DIABETIC DIET AFTER 50

Discover Over 2000 Days of Super Easy, Quick & Healthy Low-Carb, Low-Sugar Recipes with a Comprehensive 30-Day Meal Plan for Managing Type 2 Diabetes

by Moira Boyd

Copyright Notice:

Copyright © 2024 by Moira Boyd - All rights reserved.

No portion of this book may be reproduced in any form without written permission from the publisher or author, except as permitted by U.S. copyright law.

Legal Notice:

This publication is designed to provide accurate and authoritative information in regard to the subject matter covered. It is sold with the understanding that neither the author nor the publisher is engaged in rendering legal, investment, accounting or other professional services.

Disclaimer Notice:

While the publisher and author have used their best efforts in preparing this book, they make no representations or warranties with respect to the accuracy or completeness of the contents of this book and specifically disclaim any implied warranties of merchantability or fitness for a particular purpose. No warranty may be created or extended by sales representatives or written sales materials. The advice and strategies contained herein may not be suitable for your situation. You should consult with a professional when appropriate. Neither the publisher nor the author shall be liable for any loss of profit or any other commercial damages, including but not limited to special, incidental, consequential, personal, or other damages.

Table of Contents

Introduction: Your Journey to Better Health Begins Here..................5
Chapter 1: Understanding Diabetes After 50............6
The Basics of Type 2 Diabetes..................6
How Aging Affects Diabetes..................6
Key Differences from Type 1 Diabetes..................6
Chapter 2: Nutritional Foundations for Diabetics...7
The Role of Diet in Managing Type 2 Diabetes..........7
Macronutrients: What You Need to Know..................7
Micronutrients: Vitamins and Minerals Essentials....8
The Critical Role of Fiber..................9
How to Read and Understand Food Labels..................9
Chapter 3: Mastering the Diabetic Diet..................10
Creating Your Diabetic-Friendly Kitchen..................10
Shopping List Essentials: What to Buy and What to Avoid..................10
Step-by-Step Guide to Meal Planning and Prep......10
Chapter 4: Overcoming Dietary Challenges............11
Adapting to Dietary Changes: Tips and Strategies...11
Dining Out: How to Stay on Track..................12
Celebrations and Social Events: Enjoying Without Guilt..................12
Chapter 5: Recipes for a New You..................12
BREAKFAST
Energizing Starts..................13
1. Avocado Toast with Poached Egg..................13
2. Greek Yogurt with Berries..................14
3. Oatmeal with Sliced Banana and Cinnamon..........14
4. Scrambled Eggs with Spinach and Mushrooms...15
5. Rye Bread with Smoked Salmon and Cream Cheese..................15
6. Cottage Cheese with Pineapple Chunks..................16
7. Tomato and Basil Omelet..................16
BREAKFAST
Smoothie Bar..................17
8. Berry Spinach Smoothie..................17
9. Tropical Green Smoothie..................18
10. Strawberry Banana Smoothie..................18
11. Peach and Kale Smoothie..................19
12. Avocado and Berry Smoothie..................19
13. Pineapple Coconut Smoothie..................20
14. Green Apple and Kale Smoothie..................20
BREAKFAST
Warm Comforts..................21
15. Veggie-Packed Breakfast Burrito..................21
16. Apple Cinnamon Quinoa..................22
17. Zucchini Pancakes..................22
18. Savory Oatmeal with Egg and Avocado..................23
19. Warm Spiced Apples and Cottage Cheese..........23
20. Mushroom and Spinach Frittata..................24
21. Warm Cinnamon Chia Pudding..................24
LUNCH
Salads that Satisfy..................25
22. Grilled Chicken and Avocado Salad..................25
23. Apple and Walnut Spinach Salad..................26
24. Taco Salad with Ground Turkey..................26
25. Beet and Goat Cheese Salad..................27
26. Asian Chicken Salad with Sesame Dressing........27
27. Lentil and Feta Salad..................28
28. Zucchini Noodle Salad with Pesto..................28
LUNCH
Wrap It Up..................29
29. Turkey and Avocado Wrap with Spinach............29
30. Grilled Chicken Caesar Wrap..................30
31. Black Bean and Corn Salsa Wrap..................30
32. Smoked Salmon and Cream Cheese Wrap..........31
33. Falafel and Hummus Wrap with Cucumber........31
34. Buffalo Chicken and Blue Cheese Wrap..............32
35. Mediterranean Veggie Wrap with Feta..................32
LUNCH
Hearty Soups..................33
36. Creamy Cauliflower and Leek Soup..................33
37. Chicken and Quinoa Vegetable Soup..................34
38. Hearty Lentil and Spinach Soup..................34
39. Tomato Basil and Chickpea Soup..................35
40. Mushroom and Barley Soup..................35
41. Butternut Squash and Apple Soup..................36
42. Zucchini and Fresh Herb Soup..................36
DINNER
Vegetarian Ventures..................37
43. Stuffed Bell Peppers with Quinoa and Black Beans..................37

44. Eggplant Parmesan with Spinach and Ricotta...38
45. Vegetable Stir-Fry with Tofu and Broccoli.........38
46. Butternut Squash and Lentil Stew...................39
47. Cauliflower Curry with Chickpeas and Spinach 39

DINNER

Seafood Selections..40

48. Grilled Salmon with Asparagus and Lemon-Dill Sauce...................40
49. Shrimp and Quinoa Paella.................................41
50. Baked Cod with Herbed Tomatoes and Zucchini.. 41
51. Scallops with Cauliflower Mash and Garlic Spinach...................42
52. Tuna Steaks with Mango-Avocado Salsa...........42

DINNER

Poultry and Meat Plates...................................43

53. Herb-Roasted Chicken with Root Vegetables....43
54. Turkey Meatballs in Tomato Basil Sauce...........44
55. Grilled Lemon Chicken with Quinoa and Kale Salad...................44
56. Beef Stir-Fry with Bell Peppers and Snow Peas 45
57. Pork Tenderloin with Apple and Sage..................45
58. Lamb Chops with Rosemary and Garlic.............46
59. Honey Mustard Glazed Chicken Thighs.............46

DINNER

Low-Carb Comforts..47

60. Spaghetti Squash Carbonara............................47
61. Cauliflower Fried Rice with Chicken and Vegetables...................48
62. Spaghetti Squash Bolognese............................48
63. Eggplant Lasagna with Ricotta and Mozzarella.49
64. Stuffed Portobello Mushrooms with Spinach and Feta...................49
65. Cauliflower Crust Pizza with Veggie Toppings. 50
66. Chicken Alfredo with Zucchini Noodles.............50

SNACKS & SIDES

Healthy Snacks..51

67. Cucumber Slices with Hummus........................51
68. Almond and Coconut Energy Balls...................52
69. Apple Slices with Almond Butter.......................52
70. Veggie Sticks with Guacamole..........................53
71. Whole Grain Crackers with Cream Cheese........53
72. Berry and Nut Mix..54
73. Baked Zucchini Chips.......................................54

SNACKS & SIDES

Sides to Share..55

74. Garlic and Herb Roasted Brussels Sprout...........55
75. Quinoa Pilaf with Fresh Herbs..........................56
76. Cauliflower Rice with Lemon and Parsley...........56
77. Balsamic Glazed Carrots...................................57
78. Green Bean Almondine.....................................57
79. Roasted Sweet Potato Wedges.........................58
80. Garlic Parmesan Roasted Asparagus.................58

DESSERTS & SWEET TREATS

Fruit-Based Desserts.....................................59

81. Baked Apples with Cinnamon and Walnuts....... 59
82. Mixed Berry Compote with Greek Yogurt..........60
83. Grilled Peaches with Stevia and Mint.................60
84. Mango and Berry Parfait...................................61
85. Poached Pears in Red Wine..............................61
86. Tropical Fruit Salad with Lime and Coconut..... 62
87. Blueberry Chia Pudding....................................62

DESSERTS & SWEET TREATS

Diabetes-Friendly Baking..............................63

88. Almond Flour Blueberry Muffins........................63
89. Whole Wheat Banana Bread.............................64
90. Carrot and Walnut Cake with Cream Cheese Frosting...................64
91. Pumpkin Spice Bread..65
92. Oatmeal Raisin Cookies....................................65
93. Coconut Flour Brownies....................................66
94. Lemon Poppy Seed Loaf...................................66

DESSERTS & SWEET TREATS

Special Treats..67

95. Dark Chocolate Avocado Mousse.....................67
96. Raspberry and Chia Seed Pudding...................68
97. Frozen Yogurt Bark with Nuts and Berries.........68
98. Coconut Macaroons..69
99. No-Bake Chocolate Peanut Butter Bars............69
100. Matcha Green Tea Pudding.............................70
101. Strawberry Basil Sorbet...................................70

Chapter 6: Your 30-Day Meal Plan...................71

Appendix A: Glycemic Index Chart...................74

Appendix B: Micronutrient Table......................74

Appendix C: Resources for Further Reading........75

Introduction: Your Journey to Better Health Begins Here

Are you over 50 and battling Type 2 diabetes? Do you feel overwhelmed by the endless advice and complex dietary restrictions? If you're ready to take control of your health with simplicity and joy, this book is your starting point.

"Diabetic Diet After 50" is not just a cookbook; it's a comprehensive blueprint for a lifestyle transformation tailored specifically for your needs. Here, you'll discover over 2000 days of easy, quick, and nutritious recipes that will revitalize your health and simplify diabetes management.

What you can expect from this book:

- **Empowering Knowledge:** Learn why specific dietary changes are necessary and how they directly benefit your health. This book dives deep into the science of diabetes and nutrition, equipping you with the knowledge to make informed decisions.
- **Practical, Delicious Recipes:** Enjoy a variety of low-carb, low-sugar recipes that cater specifically to your dietary needs, ensuring you manage your diabetes without sacrificing flavor. From hearty breakfasts to satisfying dinners, every recipe promises delight and diversity on your plate.
- **A Comprehensive 30-Day Meal Plan:** Ease into your new dietary habits with a structured meal plan designed to simplify your daily decisions. This plan will help you steadily integrate healthier choices into your lifestyle, one delicious meal at a time.
- **Lifestyle Integration Tips:** Beyond what you eat, managing diabetes effectively involves understanding how to adjust your overall lifestyle. From dining out to dealing with social events and stress, you'll learn how to navigate challenges with ease.
- **Exclusive Resources for Long-term Success:** Gain access to indispensable tools such as a detailed Glycemic Index Chart, a comprehensive Micronutrient Table, and a curated list of Resources for Further Reading. These are designed to enhance your understanding of how different foods affect your blood sugar and overall health, providing a foundation for sustained improvements.

I'm Moira Boyd. With my professional education in diabetes management and personal experience with the condition, I understand how vital a proper diet is. I'm excited to guide you through each recipe and tip, designed to make managing your diabetes straightforward and stress-free. My goal is to help you live a richer, more active life through food that not only fuels but heals. I'm thrilled to share these insights and recipes with you, aiming to make your daily routine both healthier and more enjoyable.

By the end of this book, not only will you have a repertoire of wonderful recipes, you'll also have a deeper understanding of how to maintain stable blood sugar levels and live vibrantly.

Let's begin this journey together with the first chapter, setting the foundation for what diabetes means for you after 50 and how you can triumph over it with the right dietary approach. Prepare to transform how you eat, feel, and enjoy life, one meal at a time.

Chapter 1: Understanding Diabetes After 50

The Basics of Type 2 Diabetes

Type 2 diabetes is a chronic condition that affects the way your body metabolizes sugar (glucose), which is an essential source of energy for your body. Unlike Type 1 diabetes, where the body fails to produce insulin, Type 2 diabetes involves insulin resistance. This means your body doesn't use insulin effectively, leading to elevated blood sugar levels.

Key points:

- **Insulin Resistance:** The cells in your muscles, fat, and liver don't respond well to insulin and can't easily take up glucose from your blood.
- **High Blood Sugar Levels:** Over time, high blood sugar levels can cause severe health problems, such as heart disease, vision loss, and kidney disease.
- **Symptoms:** Increased thirst, frequent urination, unexplained weight loss, fatigue, blurred vision, and slow-healing sores.

How Aging Affects Diabetes

As you age, managing diabetes can become more challenging due to several factors:

- **Metabolic Slowdown:** As you get older, your metabolism slows down, making it harder to manage weight and blood sugar levels. This slowdown affects how your body processes food and utilizes insulin.
- **Increased Insulin Resistance:** Aging can increase insulin resistance, making it more difficult for cells to absorb glucose.
- **Muscle Mass Loss:** Loss of muscle mass, which occurs naturally with aging, can further reduce insulin sensitivity and metabolism efficiency.
- **Hormonal Changes:** Hormonal changes that occur with aging can also affect blood sugar levels and how your body responds to insulin.

Key Differences from Type 1 Diabetes

Understanding the differences between Type 1 and Type 2 diabetes is crucial for effective management:

- **Onset Age:** Type 1 diabetes is typically diagnosed in children and young adults, whereas Type 2 diabetes generally develops in adults over the age of 45.
- **Insulin Production:** In Type 1 diabetes, the body produces little to no insulin due to an autoimmune attack on the insulin-producing cells in the pancreas. In Type 2 diabetes, the body still produces insulin but is resistant to its effects.
- **Management:** Type 1 diabetes requires insulin therapy for life, while Type 2 diabetes can often be managed through diet, exercise, and medication.

Recognizing these differences aids in tailoring management strategies for Type 2 diabetes, focusing on essential lifestyle changes for older adults. With an understanding of diabetes' effects on your body, especially after 50, you can better appreciate the role of diet. The next chapter will explore the nutritional foundations for managing Type 2 diabetes, focusing on critical components of a diabetic-friendly diet. By learning about macronutrient balance and informed food choices, you'll be equipped to take control of your health and improve your quality of life.

Chapter 2: Nutritional Foundations for Diabetics

The Role of Diet in Managing Type 2 Diabetes

Diet plays a pivotal role in managing Type 2 diabetes, especially as you age. A balanced diet helps maintain stable blood sugar levels, supports weight management, and reduces the risk of diabetes-related complications. The right food choices can enhance your overall health and well-being.

Key points:

- **Blood Sugar Control:** Consuming a balanced mix of macronutrients can help keep blood sugar levels within a healthy range.
- **Weight Management:** A healthy diet can prevent weight gain, which is crucial since excess weight can increase insulin resistance.
- **Prevention of Complications:** Proper nutrition can reduce the risk of heart disease, kidney damage, and other diabetes-related complications.

Understanding the importance of diet sets the stage for making informed food choices that support your health.

Macronutrients: What You Need to Know

Macronutrients—carbohydrates, proteins, and fats—are the primary components of your diet. Each plays a unique role in your health and affects your blood sugar differently.

Carbohydrates: Selection and Impact

Carbohydrates have the most significant impact on blood sugar levels, making their selection crucial for diabetes management.

- **Complex Carbohydrates:** Found in whole grains, legumes, and vegetables, these are digested slowly, leading to a gradual increase in blood sugar levels. They are also rich in fiber, which aids in weight management and digestive health.
    - Examples: Brown rice, quinoa, lentils, and sweet potatoes.
    - . Benefits: Provide sustained energy and help maintain stable blood sugar levels.
- **Simple Carbohydrates:** Found in sugar, honey, and refined grains, these are quickly absorbed, causing rapid spikes in blood sugar.
    - Examples: White bread, pastries, and sugary drinks.
    - Drawbacks: Can lead to blood sugar spikes and are low in nutritional value.

Choosing complex carbohydrates over simple ones is essential for managing diabetes and ensuring overall health.

Proteins: Best Choices for Diabetics

Proteins are vital for repairing and building tissues and play a crucial role in maintaining muscle mass, which is important as you age.

- **Lean Proteins:** Include lean meats, poultry, fish, eggs, dairy products, legumes, and nuts.
    - Examples: Chicken breast, salmon, Greek yogurt, lentils, and almonds.
    - Benefits: Minimal impact on blood sugar and help with satiety, preventing overeating.

Incorporating a variety of lean protein sources into your diet supports muscle health and overall well-being.

Healthy Fats: What to Include and Avoid

Fats are an essential part of your diet, providing energy, supporting cell growth, and protecting organs. However, the type of fat you consume matters.

- **Healthy Fats:** Include unsaturated fats, which can improve cholesterol levels and support heart health.
    - Examples: Avocados, nuts, seeds, olive oil, and fatty fish.
    - Benefits: Promote heart health and reduce inflammation.
- **Unhealthy Fats:** Saturated and trans fats can raise cholesterol levels and increase the risk of heart disease.
    - Examples: Butter, lard, and processed foods with hydrogenated oils.
    - Drawbacks: Contribute to heart disease and other health issues.

Focusing on healthy fats while minimizing unhealthy fats is crucial for diabetes management and overall health.

Micronutrients: Vitamins and Minerals Essentials

A well-balanced diet includes essential vitamins, minerals, and antioxidants that play crucial roles in overall health and can have specific benefits for individuals with diabetes.

- **Magnesium:** Involved in glucose metabolism. Low levels are linked to insulin resistance.
    - Sources: Spinach, almonds, black beans.

- **Potassium:** Helps maintain normal blood pressure, important for heart health.
    - Sources: Bananas, sweet potatoes, spinach.

- **B Vitamins:** Support energy production and nerve function.
    - Sources: Whole grains, pork, poultry, fish, eggs.

- **Vitamin D:** Plays a role in insulin production and sensitivity.
    - Sources: Fatty fish, fortified dairy products, sunlight.

- **Vitamin E:** An antioxidant that helps protect cells and improve insulin action.
    - Sources: Almonds, sunflower seeds, spinach.

- **Chromium:** Enhances the action of insulin.
    - Sources: Broccoli, potatoes, whole grains.

- **Zinc:** Important for insulin production and immune function.
    - Sources: Oysters, beef, pumpkin seeds.

Including a variety of these nutrient-rich foods in your diet supports diabetes management and overall health.

The Critical Role of Fiber

Fiber is a crucial component of a diabetic diet, playing a significant role in managing blood sugar levels, promoting digestive health, and aiding in weight control.

- **Benefits of Fiber:**
  - Regulating Blood Sugar: Fiber, particularly soluble fiber, slows down the absorption of sugar, leading to a gradual rise in blood sugar levels.
  - Digestive Health: Adds bulk to the stool, preventing constipation and promoting regular bowel movements.
  - Feeling of Fullness: High-fiber foods tend to be more filling, helping reduce overall calorie intake.
  - Heart Health: Helps lower cholesterol levels, reduce blood pressure, and decrease the risk of heart disease.

- **Sources of Fiber:**
  - Whole Grains: Oats, barley, quinoa, brown rice.
  - Legumes: Beans, lentils, chickpeas.
  - Vegetables: Leafy greens, broccoli, carrots, Brussels sprouts.
  - Fruits: Berries, apples, pears, oranges.
  - Nuts and Seeds: Almonds, chia seeds, flaxseeds, pumpkin seeds.

Incorporating a variety of high-fiber foods into your diet supports your diabetes management and overall well-being.

How to Read and Understand Food Labels

Navigating the world of food labels can be daunting, but understanding them is crucial for making informed dietary choices.

- **Serving Size:** Check the serving size and the number of servings per container.
- **Total Carbohydrates:** Includes all forms of carbohydrates in the food.
- **Net Carbohydrates:** Subtract the grams of fiber and sugar alcohols from the total carbohydrates.
- **Added Sugars:** Look for sugars added during processing.
- **Ingredients List:** Listed in order of quantity, from highest to lowest.
- **Nutrient Content:** Focus on fiber, protein, and healthy fats.
- **Percent Daily Values (%DV):** Helps understand if a food is high or low in a particular nutrient.

By becoming proficient in reading food labels, you can make empowered choices that support your diabetes management and overall health.

Chapter 3: Mastering the Diabetic Diet

Creating a diabetic-friendly kitchen is the first step to ensuring your meals are both nutritious and delicious. By stocking your pantry with the right ingredients and equipping your kitchen with essential tools, you'll be well-prepared to make healthy eating a seamless part of your daily routine.

Creating Your Diabetic-Friendly Kitchen

Start by organizing your kitchen to make healthy cooking easier. Clear out processed foods and sugary snacks, replacing them with nutritious alternatives. Invest in kitchen tools that simplify meal preparation, such as a slow cooker, non-stick pans, and sharp knives.

Focus on having the following staples in your pantry and refrigerator:

- **Whole Grains:** Brown rice, quinoa, oats, whole wheat pasta.
- **Lean Proteins:** Chicken breast, turkey, fish, eggs, tofu, legumes.
- **Healthy Fats:** Olive oil, avocado oil, nuts, seeds.
- **Fresh Produce:** Leafy greens, berries, apples, carrots, bell peppers.
- **Low-Sugar Dairy:** Greek yogurt, low-fat milk, cheese.

Equipping your kitchen with these essentials will make it easier to prepare healthy meals that keep your blood sugar stable.

Shopping List Essentials: What to Buy and What to Avoid

Creating a comprehensive shopping list is key to staying on track with your diabetic diet. Focus on buying nutrient-dense foods while avoiding those that can spike your blood sugar levels.

To Buy:

- **Whole Grains:** Look for 100% whole wheat or whole grain labels.
- **Fresh Fruits and Vegetables:** Aim for a variety of colors and types.
- **Lean Proteins:** Choose skinless poultry, lean cuts of meat, and plant-based proteins.
- **Healthy Fats:** Opt for sources like avocados, nuts, and seeds.
- **Herbs and Spices:** Use these to flavor your food without added salt or sugar.

To Avoid:

- **Sugary Snacks:** Cookies, candies, and pastries.
- **Refined Grains:** White bread, white rice, and regular pasta.
- **Processed Foods:** Items with long ingredient lists and preservatives.
- **High-Sodium Products:** Canned soups, processed meats, and salty snacks.
- **Sugary Beverages:** Sodas, sweetened teas, and fruit juices.

By focusing on these guidelines, you can create a shopping list that supports your health goals and helps you manage your diabetes effectively.

Step-by-Step Guide to Meal Planning and Prep

Meal planning and preparation are crucial for maintaining a healthy diet, especially when managing diabetes. By planning your meals in advance, you can ensure a balanced intake of nutrients and avoid the temptation of unhealthy options.

- **Plan Your Meals:**
  - Create a weekly meal plan that includes breakfast, lunch, dinner, and snacks.
  - Focus on including a variety of foods to ensure you get a range of nutrients.
  - Make sure each meal contains a balance of protein, complex carbohydrates, and healthy fats.
- **Prepare Ingredients in Advance:**
  - Wash and chop vegetables as soon as you bring them home.
  - Cook grains and proteins in bulk and store them in the refrigerator for quick meals.
  - Portion out snacks like nuts, seeds, and fruit for easy access.
- **Cook Efficiently:**
  - Use time-saving kitchen tools like slow cookers and pressure cookers.
  - Prepare one-pot meals to minimize cleanup and simplify cooking.
  - Double recipes and freeze half for future meals.
- **Stay Flexible:**
  - Be prepared to adjust your meal plan based on your schedule and preferences.
  - Keep healthy, easy-to-prepare options on hand for days when you need something quick.

By following these steps, you can streamline your meal preparation process and ensure that you always have healthy, diabetes-friendly meals ready to go.

Remember, you are not alone in this journey. **At the end of this book, you will find a comprehensive 30-day meal plan prepared and assembled specifically for you from the recipes in this book.**

This meal plan is designed to guide you through each day with balanced, nutritious meals, empowering you to take control of your health and manage your diabetes effectively. With these tools at your disposal, you can face each day with confidence, knowing that you are making choices that support your well-being and pave the way for a healthier, happier future. Stay motivated, and embrace this journey towards better health with optimism and determination.

Chapter 4: Overcoming Dietary Challenges

Adapting to dietary changes can be challenging, but with the right strategies, you can make the transition smoother and more sustainable. Whether you're eating out, attending social events, or simply adjusting to new eating habits, there are ways to stay on track without feeling deprived.

Adapting to Dietary Changes: Tips and Strategies

Transitioning to a diabetic-friendly diet doesn't have to be overwhelming. Start by making small, manageable changes to your eating habits and gradually build on them.

- **Introduce New Foods Gradually:** Try incorporating one new healthy food each week.
- **Find Healthy Alternatives:** Look for healthier versions of your favorite foods, such as swapping white rice for quinoa or using Greek yogurt instead of sour cream.
- **Stay Hydrated:** Drink plenty of water throughout the day to stay hydrated and help manage your appetite.

- **Be Mindful of Portion Sizes:** Use smaller plates and bowls to help control portion sizes and prevent overeating.

By taking it one step at a time, you can make lasting changes to your diet that support your health and well-being.

Dining Out: How to Stay on Track

Eating out can be challenging when managing diabetes, but with a few strategies, you can enjoy restaurant meals without compromising your health.

- **Choose Restaurants Wisely:** Opt for places that offer healthy options and are willing to accommodate dietary requests.
- **Plan Ahead:** Look at the menu online before you go and decide what you'll order.
- **Ask for Modifications:** Don't hesitate to ask for dressings on the side, grilled instead of fried, or extra vegetables instead of starchy sides.
- **Control Portion Sizes:** Consider sharing a dish, ordering a half-portion, or taking half your meal home.

These strategies can help you enjoy dining out while keeping your blood sugar levels in check.

Celebrations and Social Events: Enjoying Without Guilt

Social gatherings and celebrations often revolve around food, which can be a challenge when you're trying to manage your diet. However, with some planning, you can enjoy these events without feeling guilty.

- **Eat a Healthy Snack Beforehand:** Arriving at an event hungry can lead to overeating. Have a healthy snack before you go to curb your appetite.
- **Bring a Healthy Dish:** Offer to bring a dish to share that you know is diabetes-friendly.
- **Focus on Socializing:** Remember that gatherings are about more than just food. Focus on enjoying the company and conversation.
- **Make Mindful Choices:** Survey the food options and choose healthier items like vegetables, lean proteins, and whole grains. Enjoy small portions of your favorite treats.

By utilizing these practical tips and engaging your support network, you can create a supportive environment that helps you manage your diabetes effectively.

With these strategies in place, you are well-equipped to overcome dietary challenges and maintain a healthy lifestyle. Now, let's move on to the heart of your new dietary journey – delicious, diabetes-friendly recipes that will make managing your condition both enjoyable and sustainable.

Chapter 5: Recipes for a New You

Delicious, nutritious recipes are the heart of a successful diabetic diet. This chapter provides a wide range of recipes for every meal, ensuring variety and satisfaction. Whether you are looking for quick breakfasts, satisfying lunches, hearty dinners, or tasty snacks and desserts, you'll find something to suit your taste and nutritional needs.

BREAKFAST
Energizing Starts

Note: These recipes are designed for one serving. To accommodate more people, simply multiply the ingredients by the desired number of servings.

The words "tablespoon" and "teaspoon" have been shortened to "tbsp" and "tsp".

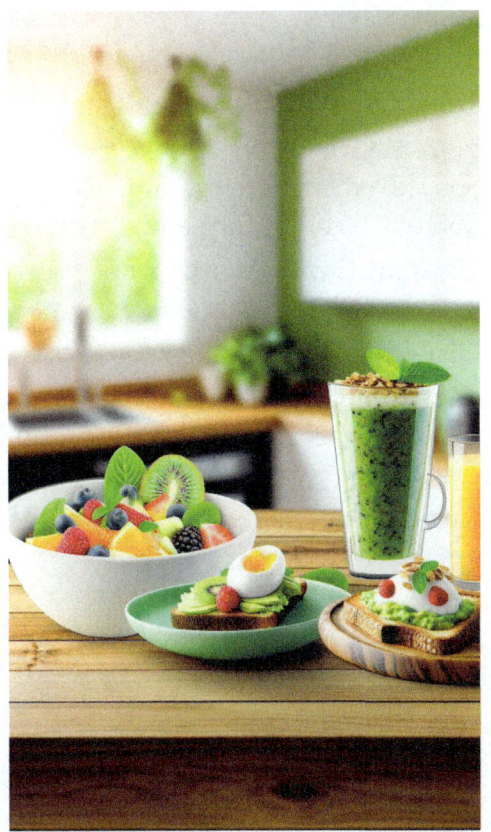

1. Avocado Toast with Poached Egg

Prep: 5 min | **Cook:** 5 min | **Total:** 10 min | **Difficulty:** 2/5

Ingredients: Whole grain bread: 1 slice (1 slice = 30g, 1.06 oz), Ripe avocado: 1 (1 avocado = 150g, 5.29 oz), Egg: 1 (1 egg = 50g, 1.76 oz), Salt and pepper: to taste

1. Preparation: Toast bread. Peel and pit the avocado, mash with a fork, and season with salt and pepper.

2. Cooking: Bring water to a simmer (around 85°C/ 185°F), crack the egg into a cup, gently lower it into the simmering water, poach for 3-4 minutes.

3. Assembly: Spread mashed avocado on toast, top with poached egg, season with additional salt and pepper if desired.

4. Serving: Garnish with fresh herbs like parsley or chives, and enjoy while the egg is warm and the toast is crisp.

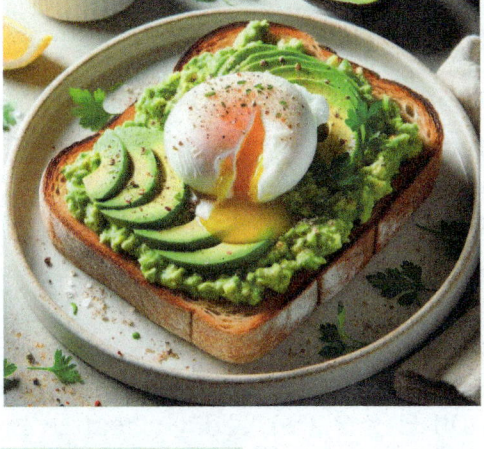

Nutritional Values: Calories: 290 kcal, Carbohydrates: 19 g, Protein: 13 g, Fat: 20 g (Saturated Fat: 4 g, Monounsaturated Fat: 10 g, Polyunsaturated Fat: 3 g), Cholesterol: 185 mg, Sodium: 360 mg, Fiber: 7 g, Sugars: 2 g

Glycemic Index: Whole grain bread: Medium (GI = 56-69), Avocado: Very Low (GI = 15), Egg: Low (GI = 0)

Chef's Tips: *"Add lemon juice/red pepper flakes to avocado, use vinegar in water for poaching egg, add arugula/spinach for extra nutrients".*

2. Greek Yogurt with Berries

Prep: 5 min | **Cook:** none | **Total:** 5 min | **Difficulty:** **1/5**

Ingredients: Plain Greek yogurt: 1 cup (245g, 8.64 oz), Mixed berries (strawberries, blueberries, raspberries): 1/2 cup (75g, 2.65 oz), Ground flaxseed: 1 tbsp (7g, 0.25 oz)

1.Preparation: Wash the berries thoroughly. If using strawberries, hull and slice them.

2.Cooking: No cooking required.

3.Assembly: Spoon the Greek yogurt into a bowl. Top with mixed berries. Sprinkle with ground flaxseed.

4.Serving: Serve immediately as a refreshing and nutritious breakfast or snack.

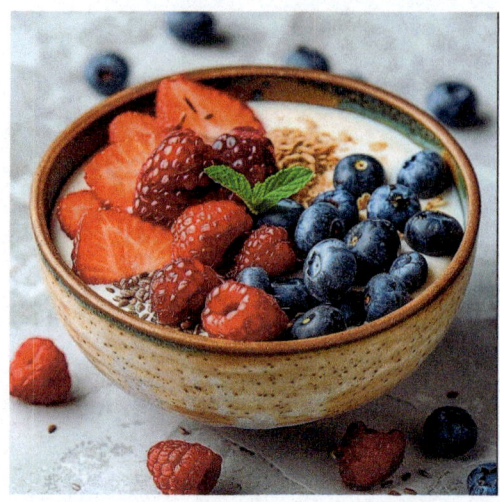

Nutritional Values: Calories: 200 kcal, Carbohydrates: 20 g, Protein: 15 g, Fat: 8 g (Saturated Fat: 4 g), Cholesterol: 20 mg, Sodium: 80 mg, Fiber: 6 g, Sugars: 12 g

Chef's Tips: *"Use a mix of fresh and frozen berries for a different texture. Add a few fresh mint leaves for a refreshing twist"*.

Glycemic Index: Greek yogurt: Low (GI = 15-30), Berries: Low (GI = 40-53), Flaxseed: Low (GI < 15)

3. Oatmeal with Sliced Banana and Cinnamon

Prep: 5 min | **Cook:** 10 min | **Total:** 15 min | **Difficulty:** **1/5**

Ingredients: Whole oat flakes: 1/2 cup (40g, 1.41 oz), Water or almond milk: 1 cup (240ml, 8.12 oz), Banana: 1 medium (118g, 4.16 oz), Cinnamon: 1/4 tsp (1g, 0.04 oz)

1.Preparation: Measure out the oat flakes and water or almond milk. Slice the banana.

2.Cooking: Combine the whole oat flakes and water or almond milk in a small saucepan, bring to a boil over medium heat (100°C / 212°F), reduce heat to low and simmer for about 10 minutes.

3.Assembly: Pour the oatmeal into a bowl. Top with sliced banana and sprinkle with cinnamon.

4.Serving: Serve immediately for a warm and comforting breakfast.

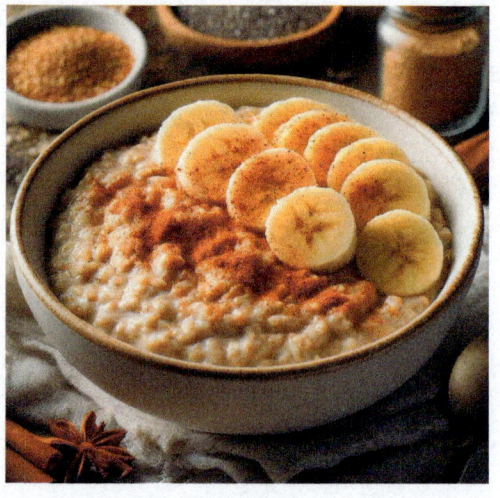

Nutritional Values: Calories: 230 kcal, Carbohydrates: 45 g, Protein: 5 g, Fat: 3 g (Saturated Fat: 0.5 g), Cholesterol: 0 mg, Sodium: 10 mg, Fiber: 7 g, Sugars: 14 g

Chef's Tips: *"Add a teaspoon of chia seeds for extra fiber, use a pinch of nutmeg for additional warmth"*.

Glycemic Index: Rolled oats: Medium (GI = 55), Banana: Medium (GI = 51), Cinnamon: Negligible GI

4. Scrambled Eggs with Spinach and Mushrooms

Prep: 3 min | **Cook:** 5 min | **Total:** 8 min | **Difficulty:** 1/5

Ingredients: Eggs: 2 (100g, 3.53 oz), Fresh spinach: 1 cup (30g, 1.06 oz), Mushrooms, sliced: 1/2 cup (35g, 1.23 oz), Olive oil: 1 tsp (5 ml), Salt and pepper: to taste

1. **Preparation:** Wash spinach and slice mushrooms.
2. **Cooking:** Heat oil in a pan, sauté mushrooms for 2 minutes. Add spinach, cook until wilted. Add beaten eggs, scramble until cooked.
3. **Assembly:** None.
4. **Serving:** Serve immediately, seasoned with salt and pepper.

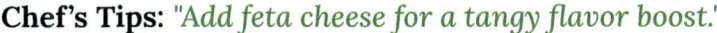

Nutritional Values: Calories: 220 kcal, Carbs: 3 g, Protein: 14 g, Fat: 17 g, Saturated Fat: 4 g, Mono Fat: 8 g, Poly Fat: 2 g, Cholesterol: 370 mg, Sodium: 320 mg, Fiber: 1 g, Sugars: 1 g

Glycemic Index: Eggs: Low (GI = 0), Spinach: Very Low (GI = 15), Mushrooms: Low (GI = 10)

Chef's Tips: *"Add feta cheese for a tangy flavor boost."*

5. Rye Bread with Smoked Salmon and Cream Cheese

Prep: 5 min | **Cook:** None | **Time:** 5 min | **Difficulty:** 1/5

Ingredients: Rye bread: 1 slice (30g, 1.06 oz), Smoked salmon: 50g (1.76 oz), Cream cheese: 2 tbsp (30g, 1.06 oz), Capers: 1 tsp (5 ml, 0.18 oz), Red onion: 2 thin slices (10g, 0.35 oz), Fresh dill: a few sprigs

1. **Preparation:** Toast the rye bread if desired. Thinly slice the red onion and wash the fresh dill.
2. **Assembly:** Spread cream cheese on the toasted rye bread. Layer with smoked salmon and red onion slices.
3. **Dressing:** Sprinkle capers over the top and garnish with fresh dill.
4. **Serving:** Serve immediately, ideally with a lemon wedge on the side for squeezing over the salmon.

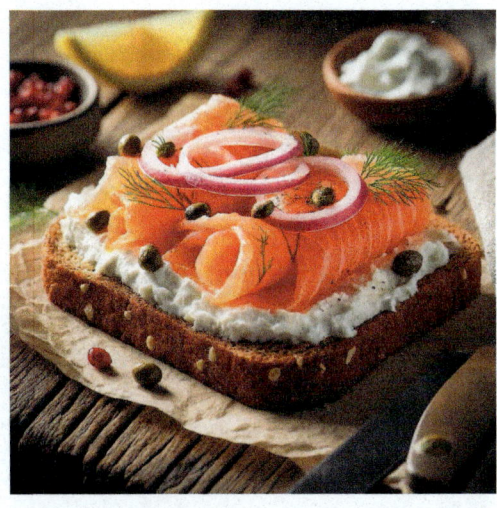

Nutritional Values: Calories: 290 kcal, Carbs: 20 g, Protein: 15 g, Fat: 16 g (Saturated Fat: 5 g, Monounsaturated Fat: 5 g, Polyunsaturated Fat: 3 g), Cholesterol: 30 mg, Sodium: 670 mg, Fiber: 3 g, Sugars: 2 g

Glycemic Index: Rye bread: Medium (GI = 56-69), Smoked salmon: Low (GI = 0), Cream cheese: Low (GI = 30)

Chef's Tips: *"For a lighter version, you can substitute cream cheese with Greek yogurt mixed with a little lemon zest."*

6. Cottage Cheese with Pineapple Chunks

Prep: 5 min | **Cook:** None | **Total:** 5 min | **Difficulty:** 1/5

Ingredients: Cottage cheese: 1 cup (225g, 7.94 oz), Pineapple chunks: 1/2 cup (75g, 2.65 oz), Fresh mint: a few leaves for garnish

1.Preparation: Cut fresh pineapple into chunks if not using pre-cut.

2.Mixing: In a bowl, combine cottage cheese and pineapple chunks.

3.Flavoring: Stir gently to combine the pineapple evenly throughout the cottage cheese.

4.Serving: Serve immediately, garnished with fresh mint leaves.

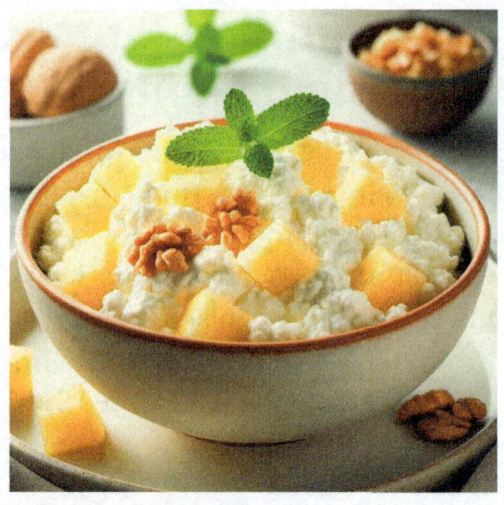

Chef's Tips: "For added crunch and flavor, sprinkle some chopped walnuts or almonds on top."

Nutritional Values: Calories: 180 kcal, Carbs: 14 g, Protein: 20 g, Fat: 5 g (Saturated Fat: 2 g, Monounsaturated Fat: 1 g, Polyunsaturated Fat: 0.5 g), Cholesterol: 15 mg, Sodium: 450 mg, Fiber: 1 g, Sugars: 12 g (natural sugars from pineapple)

Glycemic Index: Low (GI = 30), Pineapple: Medium (GI = 59)

7. Tomato and Basil Omelet

Prep: 5 min | **Cook:** 5 min | **Total:** 10 min | **Difficulty:** 2/5

Ingredients: Eggs: 2 (100g, 3.53 oz), Cherry tomatoes: 1/2 cup (75g, 2.65 oz), Fresh basil: 1/4 cup (10g, 0.35 oz), Olive oil: 1 tsp (5 ml), Salt and pepper: to taste

1.Preparation: Halve the cherry tomatoes and chop the basil.

2.Cooking: In a bowl, beat the eggs with a pinch of salt and pepper. Heat olive oil in a non-stick pan over medium heat. Pour in the eggs, cook until they start to set. Add cherry tomatoes and basil on one half of the omelet, then fold the other half over the filling. Cook for another minute until fully set.

3.Assembly: None.

4.Serving: Serve immediately, garnished with additional basil if desired.

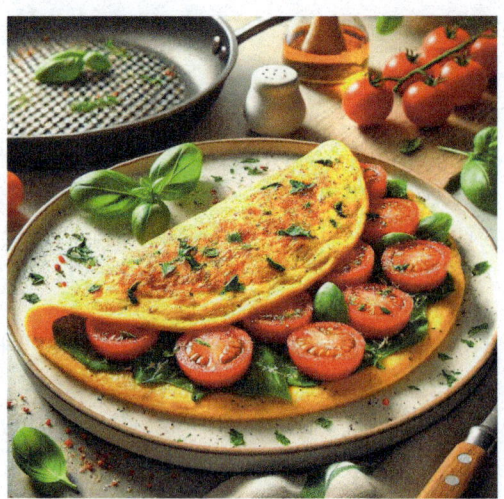

Chef's Tips: "For extra flavor, add a sprinkle of grated Parmesan cheese before folding the omelet."

Nutritional Values: Calories: 200 kcal, Carbs: 5 g, Protein: 14 g, Fat: 14 g (Saturated Fat: 3 g, Monounsaturated Fat: 8 g, Polyunsaturated Fat: 2 g), Cholesterol: 370 mg, Sodium: 300 mg, Fiber: 1 g, Sugars: 3 g

Glycemic Index: Eggs: Low (GI = 0), Tomatoes: Low (GI = 15), Basil: Very Low (GI = 5)

BREAKFAST
Smoothie Bar

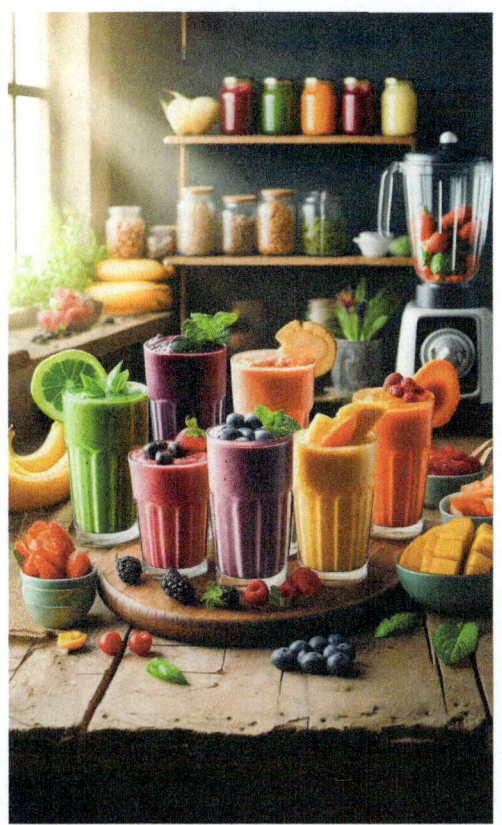

Note: These recipes are designed for one serving. To accommodate more people, simply multiply the ingredients by the desired number of servings.

The words "tablespoon" and "teaspoon" have been shortened to "tbsp" and "tsp".

8. Berry Spinach Smoothie

Prep: 5 min | **Blend:** 2 min | **Total:** 7 min | **Difficulty:** 1/5

Ingredients: Fresh spinach: 1 cup (30g, 1.06 oz), Mixed berries (strawberries, blueberries, raspberries): 1 cup (140g, 4.94 oz), Greek yogurt: 1/2 cup (123g, 4.34 oz), Almond milk: 1/2 cup (120 ml), Ice cubes: 1/2 cup

1. Preparation: Wash the spinach and berries.

2. Blending: Combine spinach, mixed berries, Greek yogurt, almond milk, and ice cubes in a blender. Blend until smooth.

3. Flavoring: If additional sweetness is desired, consider adding a small amount of stevia or another suitable sweetener for diabetics.

4. Serving: Serve immediately in a glass, garnish with a few berries.

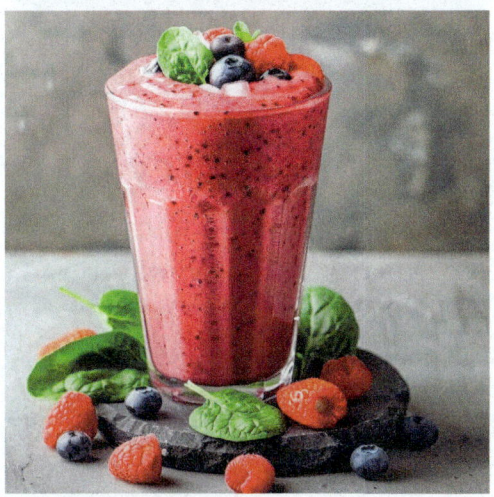

Nutritional Values: Calories: 170 kcal, Carbs: 26 g, Protein: 8 g, Fat: 4 g (Saturated Fat: 0.5 g, Monounsaturated Fat: 0.5 g, Polyunsaturated Fat: 2.5 g), Cholesterol: 5 mg, Sodium: 55 mg, Fiber: 4 g, Sugars: 16 g (natural sugars from fruits)

Glycemic Index: Spinach: Very Low (GI = 15), Berries: Low (GI = 25-40), Greek yogurt: Low (GI = 14), Almond milk: Low (GI = 25)

Chef's Tips: *"Enhance the nutritional content by adding a scoop of protein powder or a tablespoon of chia seeds to the blender."*

9. Tropical Green Smoothie

Prep: 5 min | **Blend:** 2 min | **Total:** 7 min | **Difficulty:** 1/5

Ingredients: Fresh spinach: 1 cup (30g, 1.06 oz), Pineapple chunks: 1/2 cup (75g, 2.65 oz), Mango chunks: 1/2 cup (75g, 2.65 oz), Coconut milk: 1/2 cup (120 ml), Greek yogurt: 1/2 cup (123g, 4.34 oz), Ice cubes: 1/2 cup (120 ml)

1. Preparation: Wash the spinach. Cut fresh pineapple and mango into chunks if not using pre-cut.

2. Blending: In a blender, combine spinach, pineapple chunks, mango chunks, coconut milk, Greek yogurt, and ice cubes. Blend until smooth.

3. Flavoring: Taste and adjust consistency by adding more coconut milk if desired.

4. Serving: Pour into a glass and serve immediately. Garnish with a slice of pineapple or mango on the rim of the glass if desired.

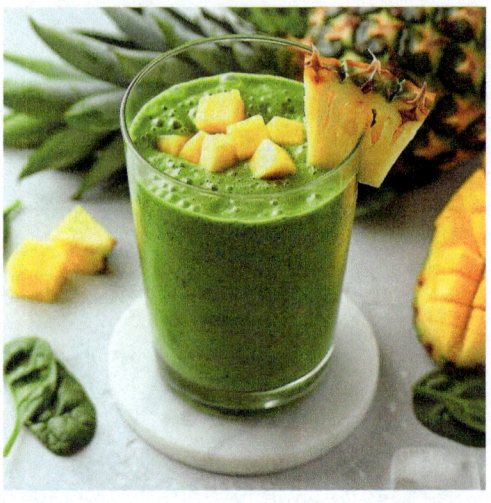

Nutritional Values: Calories: 200 kcal, Carbs: 30 g, Protein: 8 g, Fat: 7 g (Saturated Fat: 5 g, Monounsaturated Fat: 1 g, Polyunsaturated Fat: 1 g), Cholesterol: 5 mg, Sodium: 50 mg, Fiber: 4 g, Sugars: 25 g (natural sugars from fruits)

Glycemic Index: Spinach: Very Low (GI = 15), Pineapple: Medium (GI = 59), Mango: Medium (GI = 60), Coconut milk: Low (GI = 35), Greek yogurt: Low (GI = 14)

Chef's Tips: *"Add a tablespoon of chia seeds or a scoop of protein powder for an extra nutritional boost."*

10. Strawberry Banana Smoothie

Prep: 5 min | **Blend:** 2 min | **Total:** 7 min | **Difficulty:** 1/5

Ingredients: Fresh strawberries: 1 cup (150g, 5.29 oz), Banana: 1 medium (120g, 4.23 oz), Unsweetened almond milk: 1 cup (240 ml, 8.12 oz), Ice cubes: 1/2 cup (120 ml, 4.06 oz)

1. Preparation: Wash strawberries, peel bananas.

2. Blending: In a blender, combine strawberries, banana, almond milk, and ice cubes, blend until smooth.

3. Flavoring: Taste and adjust sweetness with more banana or almond milk if desired.

4. Serving: Pour into a glass, serve immediately.

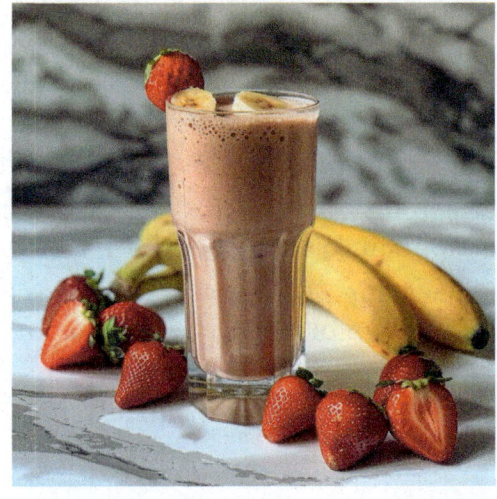

Nutritional Values: Calories: 150 kcal, Carbohydrates: 35 g, Protein: 2 g, Fat: 2 g (Saturated Fat: 0 g, Monounsaturated Fat: 0.5 g, Polyunsaturated Fat: 0.5 g), Cholesterol: 0 mg, Sodium: 60 mg, Fiber: 4 g, Sugars: 19 g

Glycemic Index: Fresh strawberries: Low (GI = 41), Banana: Medium (GI = 51), Almond milk: Low (GI = 30)

Chef's Tips: *"For added nutrition, include a tablespoon of flax seeds or a handful of spinach."*

11. Peach and Kale Smoothie

Prep: 5 min | **Blend:** 2 min | **Total:** 7 min | **Difficulty:** 1/5

Ingredients: Fresh peaches: 2 (300g, 10.58 oz), Fresh kale: 1 cup (30g, 1.06 oz), Greek yogurt: 1/2 cup (123g, 4.34 oz), Almond milk: 1/2 cup (120 ml), Ice cubes: 1/2 cup (120 ml)

1. Preparation: Wash and slice the peaches. Wash and chop the kale.

2. Blending: In a blender, combine peaches, kale, Greek yogurt, almond milk, and ice cubes. Blend until smooth.

3. Flavoring: Taste and adjust sweetness with more almond milk if desired.

4. Serving: Pour into a glass and serve immediately. Garnish with a peach slice on the rim of the glass if desired.

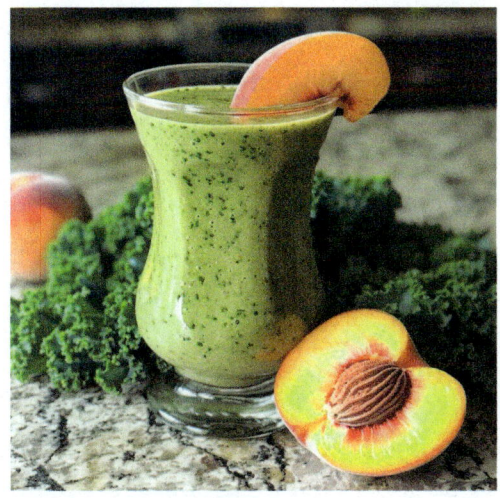

Nutritional Values: Calories: 180 kcal, Carbs: 30 g, Protein: 8 g, Fat: 4 g (Saturated Fat: 0.5 g, Monounsaturated Fat: 1 g, Polyunsaturated Fat: 2.5 g), Cholesterol: 5 mg, Sodium: 55 mg, Fiber: 5 g, Sugars: 20 g (natural sugars from fruits)

Glycemic Index: Peaches: Low (GI = 42), Kale: Very Low (GI = 15), Greek yogurt: Low (GI = 14), Almond milk: Low (GI = 25)

Chef's Tips: *"Add a tablespoon of chia seeds or a small piece of fresh ginger for an extra nutritional boost and a hint of spice."*

12. Avocado and Berry Smoothie

Prep: 5 min | **Blend:** 2 min | **Total:** 7 min | **Difficulty:** 1/5

Ingredients: Ripe avocado: 1/2 (75g, 2.65 oz), Mixed berries (strawberries, blueberries, raspberries): 1 cup (140g, 4.94 oz), Greek yogurt: 1/2 cup (123g, 4.34 oz), Almond milk: 1/2 cup (120 ml), Ice cubes: 1/2 cup (120 ml)

1. Preparation: Halve the avocado, remove the pit, and scoop out the flesh. Wash the berries.

2. Blending: In a blender, combine avocado, mixed berries, Greek yogurt, almond milk, and ice cubes. Blend until smooth.

3. Flavoring: Taste and adjust sweetness with more almond milk if desired.

4. Serving: Pour into a glass and serve immediately. Garnish with a few berries on top if desired.

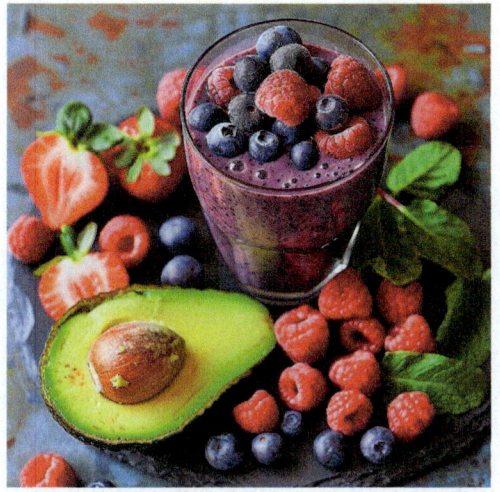

Nutritional Values: Calories: 220 kcal, Carbs: 25 g, Protein: 8 g, Fat: 12 g (Saturated Fat: 1.5 g, Monounsaturated Fat: 8 g, Polyunsaturated Fat: 2.5 g), Cholesterol: 5 mg, Sodium: 50 mg, Fiber: 7 g, Sugars: 15 g (from fruits)

Glycemic Index: Avocado: Very Low (GI = 15), Berries: Low (GI = 25-40), Greek yogurt: Low (GI = 14), Almond milk: Low (GI = 25)

Chef's Tips: *"For added nutrition, include a tablespoon of flax seeds or a handful of spinach."*

13. Pineapple Coconut Smoothie

Prep: 5 min | **Blend:** 2 min | **Total:** 7 min | **Difficulty:** 1/5

Ingredients: Pineapple chunks: 1 cup (150g, 5.29 oz), Coconut milk: 1/2 cup (120 ml), Greek yogurt: 1/2 cup (123g, 4.34 oz), Ice cubes: 1/2 cup (120 ml), Unsweetened shredded coconut: 1 tbsp (7g, 0.25 oz)

1. Preparation: Cut fresh pineapple into chunks if not using pre-cut.

2. Blending: In a blender, combine pineapple chunks, coconut milk, Greek yogurt, and ice cubes. Blend until smooth.

3. Flavoring: Taste and adjust the consistency with more coconut milk if desired.

4. Serving: Pour into a glass and serve immediately. Garnish with unsweetened shredded coconut on top.

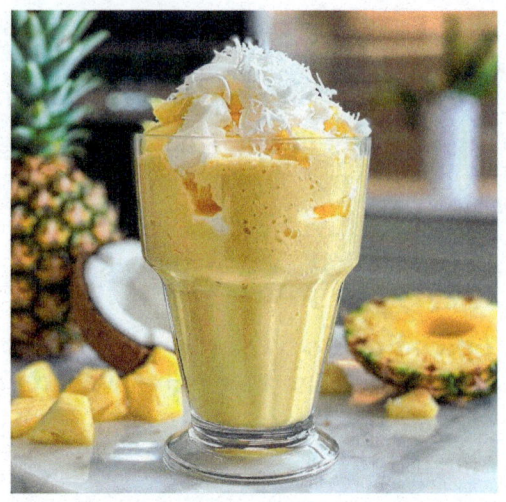

Nutritional Values: Calories: 200 kcal, Carbs: 28 g, Protein: 8 g, Fat: 7 g (Saturated Fat: 6 g, Monounsaturated Fat: 0.5 g, Polyunsaturated Fat: 0.5 g), Cholesterol: 5 mg, Sodium: 50 mg, Fiber: 3 g, Sugars: 20 g (natural sugars from pineapple)

Glycemic Index: Pineapple: Medium (GI = 59), Coconut milk: Low (GI = 35), Greek yogurt: Low (GI = 14), Unsweetened shredded coconut: Very Low (GI = 10)

Chef's Tips: *"For added flavor, include a splash of vanilla extract or a few fresh mint leaves."*

14. Green Apple and Kale Smoothie

Prep: 5 min | **Blend:** 2 min | **Total:** 7 min | **Difficulty:** 1/5

Ingredients: Green apple: 1 medium (182g, 6.42 oz), Fresh kale: 1 cup (30g, 1.06 oz), Greek yogurt: 1/2 cup (123g, 4.34 oz), Almond milk: 1/2 cup (120 ml), Ice cubes: 1/2 cup (120 ml), Lemon juice: 1 tbsp (15 ml)

1. Preparation: Wash and core the green apple, then cut into chunks. Wash and chop the kale.

2. Blending: In a blender, combine green apple chunks, kale, Greek yogurt, almond milk, ice cubes, and lemon juice. Blend until smooth.

3. Flavoring: Taste and adjust sweetness with more almond milk if desired.

4. Serving: Pour into a glass and serve immediately. Garnish with a slice of green apple or a lemon wedge on the rim of the glass if desired.

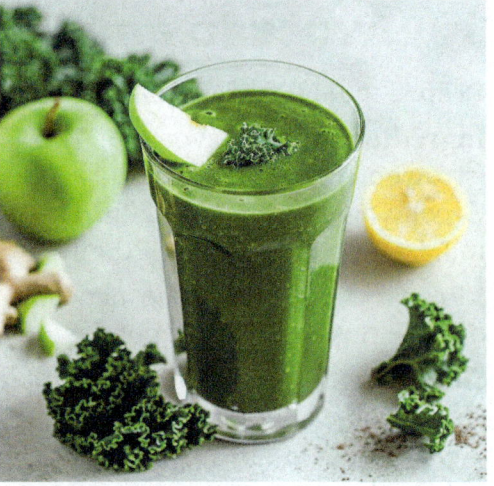

Nutritional Values: Calories: 180 kcal, Carbs: 30 g, Protein: 8 g, Fat: 4 g (Saturated Fat: 0.5 g, Monounsaturated Fat: 1 g, Polyunsaturated Fat: 2.5 g), Cholesterol: 5 mg, Sodium: 55 mg, Fiber: 5 g, Sugars: 20 g (natural sugars from fruits)

Glycemic Index: Green apple: Medium (GI = 39), Kale: Very Low (GI = 15), Greek yogurt: Low (GI = 14), Almond milk: Low (GI = 25)

Chef's Tips: *"Add a tablespoon of flax seeds or a small piece of fresh ginger for an extra nutritional boost and a hint of spice."*

BREAKFAST
Warm Comforts

Note: These recipes are designed for one serving. To accommodate more people, simply multiply the ingredients by the desired number of servings.

The words "tablespoon" and "teaspoon" have been shortened to "tbsp" and "tsp".

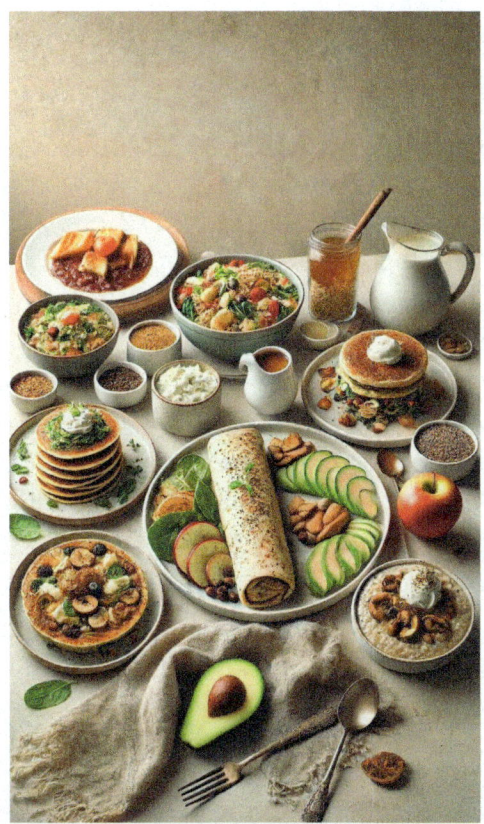

15. Veggie-Packed Breakfast Burrito

Prep: 10 min | **Cook:** 10 min | **Total:** 20 min | **Difficulty:** 2/5

Ingredients: Whole wheat tortilla: 1 large (60g, 2.12 oz), Eggs: 2 (100g, 3.53 oz), Olive oil: 1 tsp (5 ml), Red bell pepper: 1/2 cup (75g, 2.65 oz), Spinach: 1 cup (30g, 1.06 oz), Black beans: 1/4 cup (60g, 2.12 oz), Cheddar cheese, shredded: 1/4 cup (30g, 1.06 oz), Salsa: 2 tbsp (30g, 1.06 oz), Salt and pepper: to taste

1. Preparation: Dice the red bell pepper and wash the spinach.

2. Cooking: Heat olive oil in a pan over medium heat. Sauté bell pepper for 3-4 minutes until softened. Add spinach and cook until wilted. In a bowl, beat the eggs with a pinch of salt and pepper, then pour into the pan with the vegetables. Scramble until eggs are fully cooked.

3. Assembly: Warm the tortilla in a separate pan or microwave. Place scrambled eggs with vegetables on the tortilla, add black beans, shredded cheddar cheese, and salsa.

4. Serving: Roll the tortilla into a burrito and serve immediately.

Chef's Tips: *"For added flavor, include a slice of avocado or a dollop of Greek yogurt inside the burrito."*

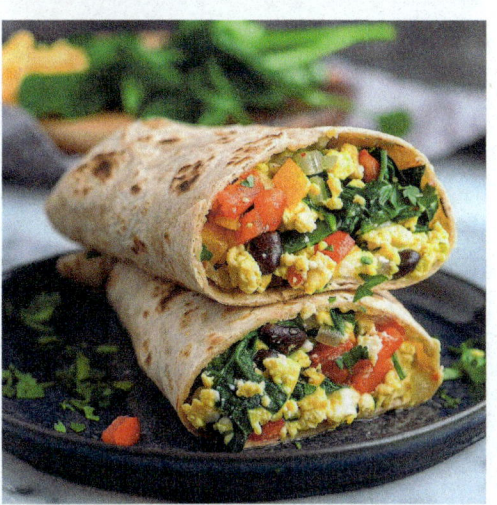

Nutritional Values: Calories: 350 kcal, Carbs: 30 g, Protein: 20 g, Fat: 18 g (Saturated Fat: 6 g, Monounsaturated Fat: 8 g, Polyunsaturated Fat: 2 g), Cholesterol: 380 mg, Sodium: 600 mg, Fiber: 6 g, Sugars: 4 g

Glycemic Index: Whole wheat tortilla: Medium (GI = 50), Eggs: Low (GI = 0), Bell pepper: Low (GI = 15), Spinach: Very Low (GI = 15), Black beans: Low (GI = 30), Cheddar cheese: Low (GI = 30), Salsa: Low (GI = 30)

16. Apple Cinnamon Quinoa

Prep: 5 min | **Cook**: 15 min | **Total**: 20 min | **Difficulty**: 2/5

Ingredients: Quinoa: 1/2 cup (85g, 3 oz), Water: 1 cup (240 ml), Apple: 1 medium (182g, 6.42 oz), Ground cinnamon: 1 tsp (2.5g, 0.09 oz), Almond milk: 1/2 cup (120 ml), Walnuts, chopped: 2 tbsp (15g, 0.53 oz), Stevia: to taste

1. Preparation: Rinse the quinoa under cold water. Core and dice the apple.

2. Cooking: In a saucepan, bring water to a boil. Add quinoa, reduce heat, cover, and simmer for 15 minutes or until quinoa is tender and water is absorbed. In the last 5 minutes of cooking, stir in the diced apple and cinnamon.

3. Mixing: Remove from heat and stir in almond milk and stevia to taste.

4. Serving: Divide the quinoa mixture into bowls, top with chopped walnuts, and serve warm.

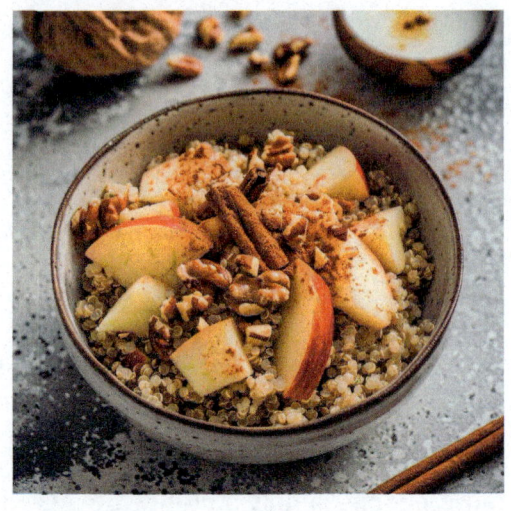

Nutritional Values: Calories: 280 kcal, Carbs: 46 g, Protein: 7 g, Fat: 9 g (Saturated Fat: 0.5 g, Monounsaturated Fat: 2 g, Polyunsaturated Fat: 5 g), Cholesterol: 0 mg, Sodium: 20 mg, Fiber: 6 g, Sugars: 12 g (natural sugars from apple)

Glycemic Index: Quinoa: Low (GI = 53), Apple: Medium (GI = 39), Cinnamon: Very Low (GI = 5), Almond milk: Low (GI = 25), Walnuts: Very Low (GI = 15)

Chef's Tips: *"For extra flavor, add a dash of vanilla extract or a sprinkle of nutmeg."*

17. Zucchini Pancakes

Prep: 10 min | **Cook**: 15 min | **Total**: 25 min | **Difficulty**: 2/5

Ingredients: Zucchini: 2 medium (400g, 14.1 oz), Eggs: 2 (100g, 3.53 oz), Whole wheat flour: 1/2 cup (60g, 2.12 oz), Green onions, chopped: 1/4 cup (30g, 1.06 oz), Garlic, minced: 2 cloves (6g, 0.21 oz), Olive oil: 2 tbsp (30 ml, 1.01 oz), Salt and pepper: to taste, Greek yogurt: 1/2 cup (123g, 4.34 oz) for serving

1. Preparation: Grate the zucchini and squeeze out excess moisture using a clean kitchen towel. Chop the green onions and mince the garlic.

2. Mixing: In a large bowl, combine grated zucchini, eggs, whole wheat flour, chopped green onions, and minced garlic. Season with salt and pepper and mix until well combined.

3. Cooking: Heat olive oil in a non-stick skillet over medium heat. Scoop about 1/4 cup of the batter for each pancake into the skillet, flattening slightly. Cook for 3-4 minutes on each side until golden brown and cooked through.

4. Serving: Serve warm with a dollop of Greek yogurt on top.

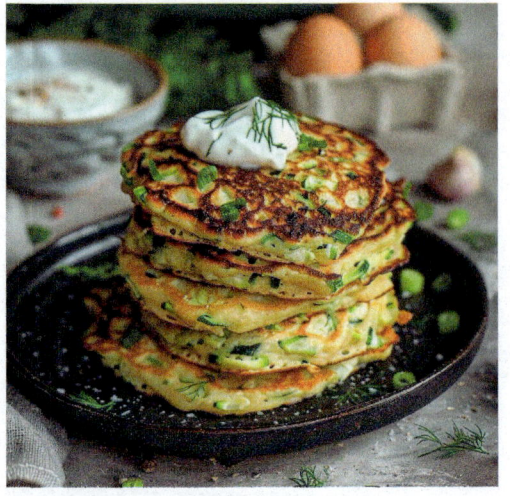

Nutritional Values: Calories: 250 kcal, Carbs: 20 g, Protein: 10 g, Fat: 15 g (Saturated Fat: 3 g, Monounsaturated Fat: 8 g, Polyunsaturated Fat: 2 g), Cholesterol: 110 mg, Sodium: 200 mg, Fiber: 3 g, Sugars: 5 g

Glycemic Index: Zucchini: Very Low (GI = 15), Whole wheat flour: Medium (GI = 69), Eggs: Low (GI = 0), Greek yogurt: Low (GI = 14)

Chef's Tips: *"For added flavor, mix some chopped fresh herbs like dill or parsley into the batter."*

18. Savory Oatmeal with Egg and Avocado

Prep: 5 min | **Cook:** 10 min | **Total:** 15 min | **Difficulty:** 2/5

Ingredients: Rolled oats: 1/2 cup (45g, 1.59 oz), Water: 1 cup (240 ml), Egg: 1 large (50g, 1.76 oz), Avocado: 1/2 medium (75g, 2.65 oz), Cherry tomatoes: 1/4 cup (37.5g, 1.32 oz), Olive oil: 1 tsp (5 ml), Salt and pepper: to taste, Fresh herbs (optional): 1 tbsp, chopped

1.Preparation: Halve the avocado and scoop out the flesh. Slice the cherry tomatoes.

2.Cooking: In a small saucepan, bring water to a boil. Add rolled oats and reduce heat, simmer for about 5 minutes, stirring occasionally. In another pan, heat olive oil and fry the egg until the white is set but the yolk is still runny, about 3-4 minutes.

3.Assembly: Spoon the cooked oatmeal into a bowl. Top with fried egg, avocado slices, and cherry tomatoes.

4.Serving: Season with salt and pepper, and garnish with fresh herbs if desired. Serve immediately.

Chef's Tips: *"For an extra kick, sprinkle some red pepper flakes or a drizzle of hot sauce."*

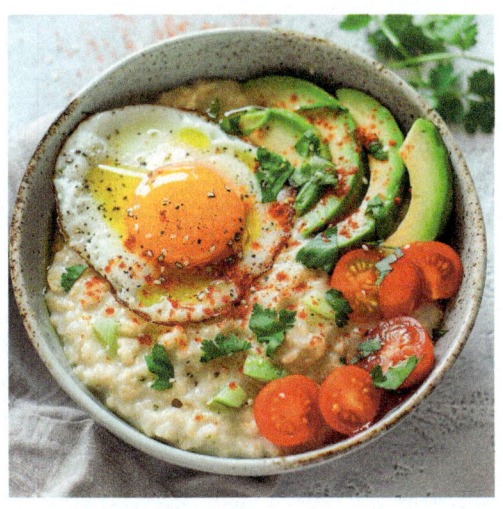

Nutritional Values: Calories: 300 kcal, Carbs: 30 g, Protein: 12 g, Fat: 15 g (Saturated Fat: 3 g, Monounsaturated Fat: 8 g, Polyunsaturated Fat: 2 g), Cholesterol: 210 mg, Sodium: 200 mg, Fiber: 8 g, Sugars: 2 g

Glycemic Index: Rolled oats: Medium (GI = 55-70), Egg: Low (GI = 0), Avocado: Very Low (GI = 15), Cherry tomatoes: Low (GI = 15)

19. Warm Spiced Apples and Cottage Cheese

Prep: 5 min | **Cook:** 10 min | **Total:** 15 min | **Difficulty:** 1/5

Ingredients: Apple: 1 medium (182g, 6.42 oz), Cottage cheese: 1 cup (225g, 7.94 oz), Ground cinnamon: 1 tsp (2.5g, 0.09 oz), Nutmeg: 1/4 tsp (0.6g, 0.02 oz), Water: 1/4 cup (60 ml), Stevia: to taste

1.Preparation: Core and slice the apple.

2.Cooking: In a small saucepan, combine apple slices, water, ground cinnamon, and nutmeg. Cook over medium heat for about 10 minutes until apples are tender, stirring occasionally.

3.Mixing: Remove from heat and stir in stevia to taste.

4.Serving: Spoon warm spiced apples over cottage cheese and serve immediately.

Chef's Tips: *"For added texture, sprinkle with chopped nuts or seeds."*

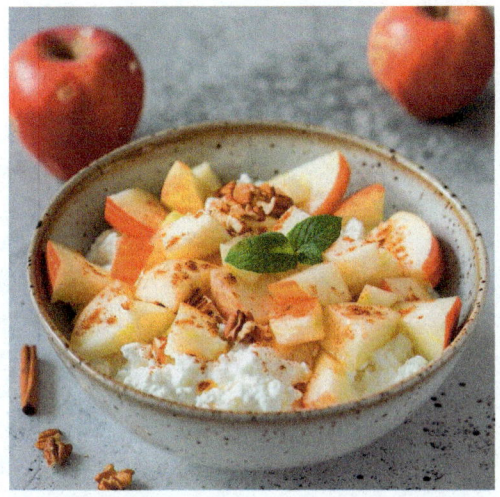

Nutritional Values: Calories: 180 kcal, Carbs: 20 g, Protein: 14 g, Fat: 5 g (Saturated Fat: 2.5 g, Monounsaturated Fat: 1 g, Polyunsaturated Fat: 0.5 g), Cholesterol: 15 mg, Sodium: 450 mg, Fiber: 4 g, Sugars: 15g (from the apple)

Glycemic Index: Apple: Medium (GI = 39), Cottage cheese: Low (GI = 30), Cinnamon: Very Low (GI = 5), Nutmeg: Very Low (GI = 5)

20. Mushroom and Spinach Frittata

Prep: 10 min | **Cook:** 15 min | **Total:** 25 min | **Difficulty:** 2/5

Ingredients: Eggs: 4 (200g, 7.05 oz), Fresh spinach: 2 cups (60g, 2.12 oz), Mushrooms, sliced: 1 cup (70g, 2.47 oz), Onion, chopped: 1/2 cup (75g, 2.65 oz), Olive oil: 2 tbsp (30 ml), Salt and pepper: to taste, Parmesan cheese, grated: 1/4 cup (25g, 0.88 oz)

1. Preparation: Chop spinach, slice mushrooms, chop onion.

2. Cooking: Heat oil in an oven-safe skillet. Sauté onion 3-4 min. Add mushrooms, cook for 5 min. Add spinach, cook until wilted. Beat eggs with salt and pepper, pour into skillet. Cook 2-3 min.

3. Baking: Preheat broiler. Sprinkle cheese on top, broil 3-5 min until golden.

4. Serving: Cool slightly, slice, serve warm.

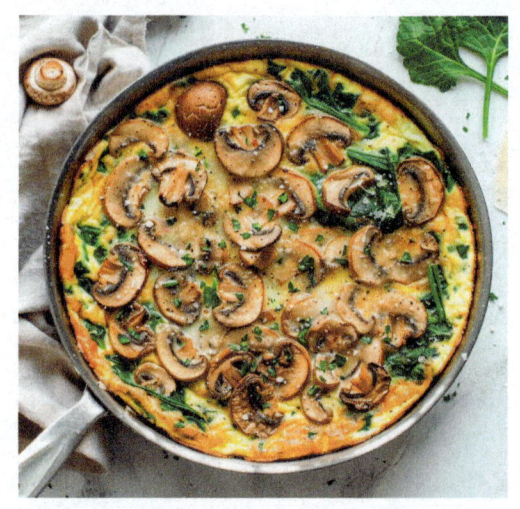

Nutritional Values: Calories: 320 kcal, Carbs: 8 g, Protein: 22 g, Fat: 24 g (Saturated Fat: 6 g, Monounsaturated Fat: 12 g, Polyunsaturated Fat: 3 g), Cholesterol: 600 mg, Sodium: 450 mg, Fiber: 2 g, Sugars: 3 g

Glycemic Index: Eggs: Low (GI = 0), Spinach: Very Low (GI = 15), Mushrooms: Low (GI = 10), Onion: Low (GI = 10), Parmesan cheese: Low (GI = 30)

Chef's Tips: *"For added flavor, mix in some fresh herbs like parsley or chives before baking."*

21. Warm Cinnamon Chia Pudding

Prep: 5 min | **Cook:** 10 min | **Total:** 15 min | **Difficulty:** 1/5

Ingredients: Chia seeds: 1/4 cup (40g, 1.41 oz), Almond milk: 1 cup (240 ml), Water: 1/2 cup (120 ml), Ground cinnamon: 1 tsp (2.5g, 0.09 oz), Vanilla extract: 1/2 tsp (2.5 ml), Stevia: to taste, Fresh berries: 1/4 cup (37.5g, 1.32 oz) for topping

1. Preparation: Combine chia seeds, almond milk, water, ground cinnamon, vanilla extract, and stevia in a saucepan.

2. Cooking: Heat the mixture over medium heat, stirring frequently until it begins to thicken, about 8-10 minutes.

3. Mixing: Once thickened, remove from heat and let it sit for a few minutes to continue absorbing liquid.

4. Serving: Spoon the warm chia pudding into bowls and top with fresh berries. Serve immediately.

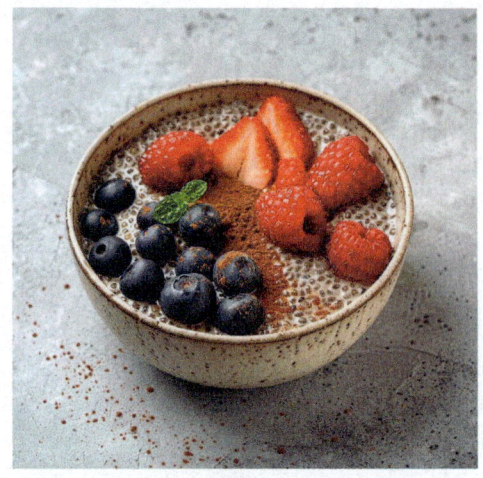

Nutritional Values: Calories: 150 kcal, Carbs: 18 g, Protein: 5 g, Fat: 7 g (Saturated Fat: 0.5 g, Monounsaturated Fat: 1.5g, Polyunsaturated Fat: 4 g), Cholesterol: 0mg, Sodium: 50mg, Fiber: 10g, Sugars: 3g

Glycemic Index: Chia seeds: Very Low (GI = 1), Almond milk: Low (GI = 25), Cinnamon: Very Low (GI = 5), Berries: Low (GI = 25-40)

Chef's Tips: *"For added crunch, sprinkle some chopped nuts or seeds on top before serving."*

LUNCH
Salads that Satisfy

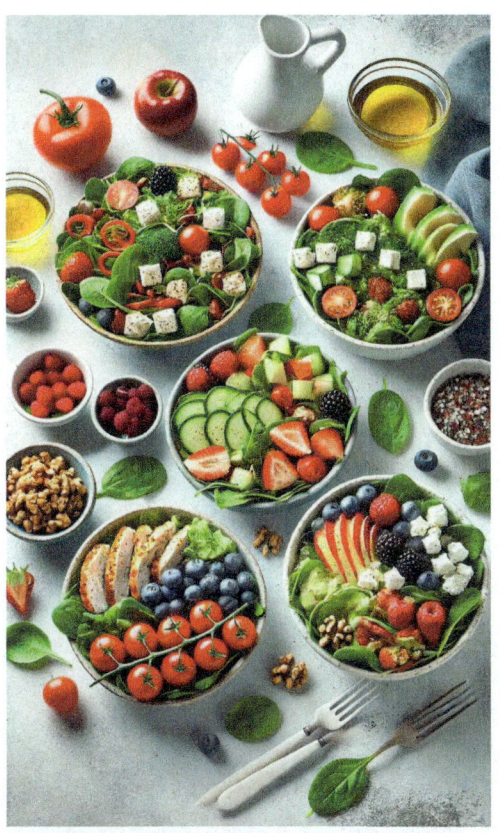

Note: These recipes are designed for one serving. To accommodate more people, simply multiply the ingredients by the desired number of servings.

The words "tablespoon" and "teaspoon" have been shortened to "tbsp" and "tsp".

22. Grilled Chicken and Avocado Salad

Prep: 10 min | **Cook:** 10 min | **Total:** 20 min | **Difficulty:** 2/5

Ingredients: Chicken breast: 150g (5.29 oz), Olive oil: 1 tbsp (15 ml, 0.51 oz), Salt and pepper: to taste, Mixed greens: 2 cups (60g, 2.12 oz), Avocado: 1/2 (75g, 2.65 oz), Cherry tomatoes: 1/2 cup (75g, 2.65 oz), Cucumber: 1/2 cup (60g, 2.12 oz), Lemon juice: 1 tbsp (15 ml, 0.51 oz)

1. **Preparation:** Season chicken with olive oil, salt, and pepper. Slice avocado, cherry tomatoes, and cucumber.
2. **Cooking:** Grill chicken over medium heat (180°C / 350°F) for 6-7 minutes on each side until fully cooked. Let rest for a few minutes, then slice.
3. **Mixing:** In a large bowl, combine mixed greens, cherry tomatoes, cucumber, and avocado.
4. **Dressing:** Drizzle with lemon juice, toss gently.
5. **Serving:** Top salad with grilled chicken slices, serve immediately.

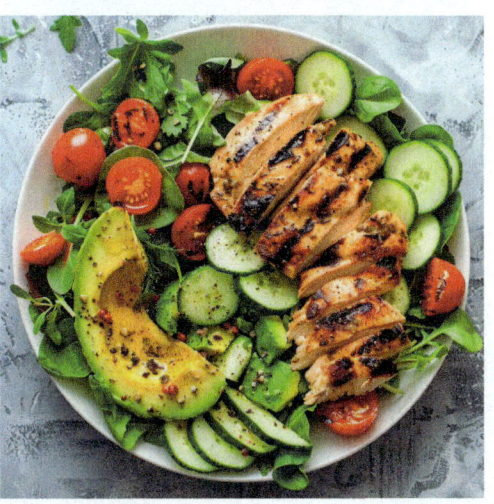

Nutritional Values: Calories: 350 kcal, Carbs: 12 g, Protein: 30 g, Fat: 20 g (Saturated Fat: 3 g, Monounsaturated Fat: 12 g, Polyunsaturated Fat: 2 g), Cholesterol: 70 mg, Sodium: 400 mg, Fiber: 6 g, Sugars: 2 g

Glycemic Index: Chicken breast: Low (GI = 0), Mixed greens: Very Low (GI = 5), Avocado: Very Low (GI = 15), Cherry tomatoes: Low (GI = 15), Cucumber: Very Low (GI = 15)

Chef's Tips: *"Add a sprinkle of cheese or nuts for extra flavor."*

23. Apple and Walnut Spinach Salad

Prep: 10 min | **Total:** 10 min | **Difficulty:** 1/5

Ingredients: Fresh spinach: 2 cups (60g, 2.12 oz), Apple: 1 medium (182g, 6.42 oz), Walnuts, chopped: 1/4 cup (30g, 1.06 oz), Red onion, thinly sliced: 1/4 cup (37.5g, 1.32 oz), Olive oil: 2 tbsp (30 ml, 1.01 oz), Balsamic vinegar: 1 tbsp (15 ml, 0.51 oz), Salt and pepper: to taste

1. **Preparation:** Wash and dry the spinach. Core and thinly slice the apple. Thinly slice the red onion.
2. **Mixing:** In a large bowl, combine spinach, apple slices, chopped walnuts, and red onion.
3. **Dressing:** In a small bowl, whisk together olive oil, balsamic vinegar, salt, and pepper. Drizzle over the salad and toss gently.
4. **Serving:** Serve immediately.

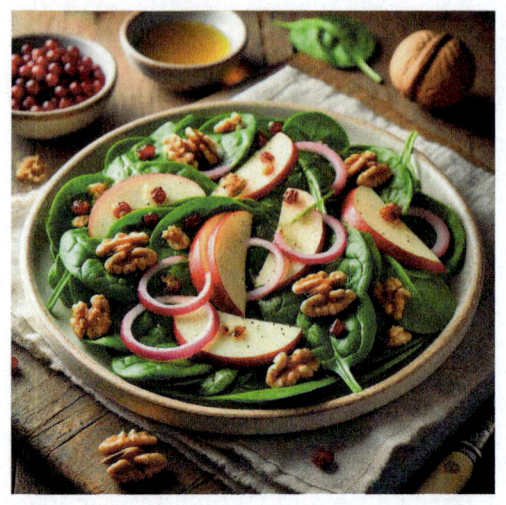

Nutritional Values: Calories: 250 kcal, Carbs: 20 g, Protein: 4 g, Fat: 18 g (Saturated Fat: 2 g, Monounsaturated Fat: 12 g, Polyunsaturated Fat: 3 g), Cholesterol: 0 mg, Sodium: 100 mg, Fiber: 5 g, Sugars: 11 g

Glycemic Index: Spinach: Very Low (GI = 15), Apple: Medium (GI = 39), Walnuts: Very Low (GI = 15), Onion: Low (GI = 10)

Chef's Tips: *"For added sweetness, you can include a handful of dried cranberries (without added sugar)."*

24. Taco Salad with Ground Turkey

Prep: 10 min | **Cook:** 15 min | **Total:** 25 min | **Difficulty:** 2/5

Ingredients: Ground turkey: 200g (7.05 oz), Olive oil: 1 tbsp (15 ml, 0.51 oz), Taco seasoning: 1 tbsp (15g, 0.53 oz), Romaine lettuce: 2 cups (60g, 2.12 oz), Cherry tomatoes: 1/2 cup (75g, 2.65 oz), Black beans: 1/2 cup (130g, 4.59 oz), Corn kernels: 1/2 cup (75g, 2.65 oz), Avocado: 1/2 (75g, 2.65 oz), Cheddar cheese, shredded: 1/4 cup (30g, 1.06 oz), Lime juice: 1 tbsp (15 ml, 0.51 oz), Salt and pepper: to taste

1. **Preparation:** Wash and chop the romaine lettuce. Halve the cherry tomatoes. Dice the avocado.
2. **Cooking:** Heat olive oil in a pan over medium heat. Add ground turkey and cook until browned. Stir in taco seasoning and cook for another 2 minutes.
3. **Assembly:** In a large bowl, combine romaine lettuce, cherry tomatoes, black beans, corn kernels, avocado, and cooked turkey. Sprinkle shredded cheddar cheese on top.
4. **Serving:** Drizzle with lime juice, season with salt and pepper, and serve immediately.

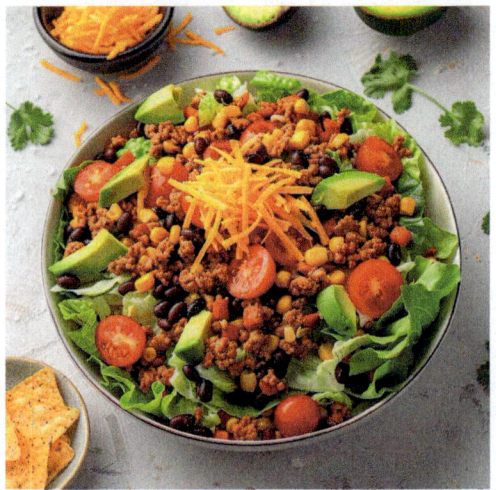

Nutritional Values: Calories: 450 kcal, Carbs: 30 g, Protein: 30 g, Fat: 25 g (Saturated Fat: 8 g, Monounsaturated Fat: 10 g, Polyunsaturated Fat: 5 g), Cholesterol: 90 mg, Sodium: 600 mg, Fiber: 10 g, Sugars: 5 g

Glycemic Index: Ground turkey: Low (GI = 0), Romaine lettuce: Very Low (GI = 5), Cherry tomatoes: Low (GI = 15), Black beans: Low (GI = 30), Corn kernels: Medium (GI = 60), Avocado: Very Low (GI = 15), Cheddar cheese: Low (GI = 30)

Chef's Tips: *"For added crunch, top with a few crushed tortilla chips or serve with a side of salsa."*

25. Beet and Goat Cheese Salad

Prep: 10 min | **Cook:** 30 min | **Total:** 40 min | **Difficulty:** 3/5
Ingredients: Beets: 2 medium (200g, 7.05 oz), Goat cheese: 1/4 cup (60g, 2.12 oz), Mixed greens: 2 cups (60g, 2.12 oz), Walnuts, chopped: 1/4 cup (30g, 1.06 oz), Olive oil: 2 tbsp (30 ml, 1.01 oz), Balsamic vinegar: 1 tbsp (15 ml, 0.51 oz), Salt and pepper: to taste

1. **Preparation:** Preheat the oven to 200°C (400°F). Wash the beets, wrap them in foil, and roast for 30 minutes or until tender. Let cool, then peel and dice.
2. **Mixing:** In a large bowl, combine mixed greens, roasted beets, and crumbled goat cheese.
3. **Dressing:** In a small bowl, whisk together olive oil, balsamic vinegar, salt, and pepper. Drizzle over the salad and toss gently to combine.
4. **Serving:** Sprinkle walnuts on top and serve immediately.

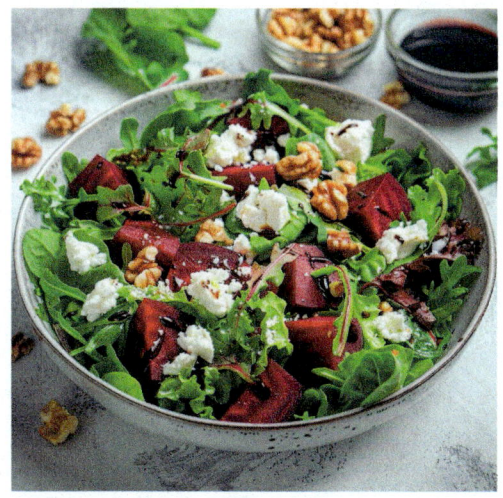

Nutritional Values: Calories: 350 kcal, Carbs: 20 g, Protein: 10 g, Fat: 26 g (Saturated Fat: 6 g, Monounsaturated Fat: 16 g, Polyunsaturated Fat: 4 g), Cholesterol: 15 mg, Sodium: 300 mg, Fiber: 6 g, Sugars: 10 g
Glycemic Index: Beets: Medium (GI = 64), Goat cheese: Low (GI = 30), Mixed greens: Very Low (GI = 5), Walnuts: Very Low (GI = 15)

Chef's Tips: *"For added flavor, toast the walnuts lightly in a dry pan before adding them to the salad."*

26. Asian Chicken Salad with Sesame Dressing

Prep: 15 min | **Cook:** 10 min | **Total:** 25 min | **Difficulty:** 2/5
Ingredients: Chicken breast: 150g (5.29 oz), Olive oil: 1 tbsp (15 ml, 0.51 oz), Salt and pepper: to taste, Mixed greens: 2 cups (60g, 2.12 oz), Red cabbage, shredded: 1 cup (70g, 2.47 oz), Carrot, julienned: 1/2 cup (60g, 2.12 oz), Cucumber, sliced: 1/2 cup (60g, 2.12 oz), Green onions, chopped: 1/4 cup (30g, 1.06 oz), Sesame seeds: 1 tbsp (15g, 0.53 oz)
Sesame Dressing: Soy sauce: 1 tbsp (15 ml, 0.51 oz), Rice vinegar: 1 tbsp (15 ml, 0.51 oz), Sesame oil: 1 tsp (5 ml, 0.18 oz), Fresh ginger, grated: 1 tsp (5g, 0.18 oz), Stevia: to taste

1. **Preparation:** Season chicken with olive oil, salt, and pepper. Prepare vegetables: shred cabbage, julienne carrot, slice cucumber, chop green onions.
2. **Cooking:** Grill chicken over medium heat (180°C / 350°F) for 6-7 minutes on each side until fully cooked. Let rest, then slice.
3. **Mixing:** Combine mixed greens, red cabbage, carrot, cucumber, and green onions in a bowl.
4. **Dressing:** Whisk together soy sauce, rice vinegar, sesame oil, grated ginger, and stevia. Drizzle over salad and toss gently.
5. **Serving:** Top with sliced chicken and sesame seeds.

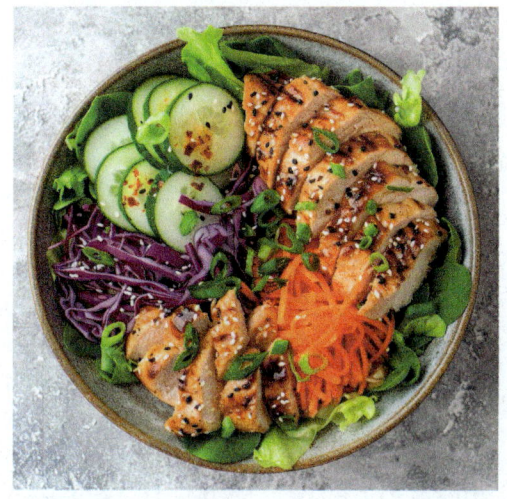

Nutritional Values: Calories: 320 kcal, Carbs: 18 g, Protein: 28 g, Fat: 16 g (Saturated Fat: 2 g, Monounsaturated Fat: 8 g, Polyunsaturated Fat: 5 g), Cholesterol: 60 mg, Sodium: 600 mg, Fiber: 6 g, Sugars: 4 g

Glycemic Index: Chicken breast: Low (GI = 0), Mixed greens: Very Low (GI = 5), Red cabbage: Very Low (GI = 15), Carrot: Low (GI = 35), Cucumber: Very Low (GI = 15)

Chef's Tips: *"For added crunch, include chopped peanuts or cashews."*

27. Lentil and Feta Salad

Prep: 10 min | **Cook:** 20 min | **Total:** 30 min | **Difficulty:** 2/5

Ingredients: Lentils: 1 cup (200g, 7.05 oz), Water: 2 cups (480 ml), Feta cheese, crumbled: 1/2 cup (75g, 2.65 oz), Cherry tomatoes, halved: 1 cup (150g, 5.29 oz), Cucumber, diced: 1 cup (120g, 4.23 oz), Red onion, finely chopped: 1/4 cup (37.5g, 1.32 oz), Fresh parsley, chopped: 1/4 cup (15g, 0.53 oz), Olive oil: 2 tbsp (30 ml, 1.01 oz), Lemon juice: 2 tbsp (30 ml, 1.01 oz), Salt and pepper: to taste

1. **Preparation:** Rinse the lentils under cold water.
2. **Cooking:** In a medium saucepan, combine lentils and water. Bring to a boil, then reduce heat and simmer for 20 minutes or until lentils are tender. Drain and let cool.
3. **Mixing:** In a large bowl, combine cooked lentils, cherry tomatoes, cucumber, red onion, and parsley.
4. **Dressing:** Whisk together olive oil, lemon juice, salt, and pepper. Drizzle over salad and toss gently to combine.
5. **Serving:** Top with crumbled feta cheese and serve.

Chef's Tips: *"For extra flavor and texture, add some chopped olives or toasted seeds. You can also include some chopped fresh mint or cilantro for added freshness."*

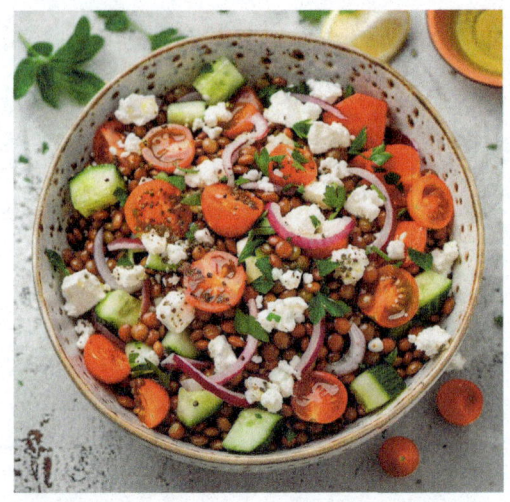

Nutritional Values: Calories: 320 kcal, Carbs: 36 g, Protein: 14 g, Fat: 14 g (Saturated Fat: 4 g, Monounsaturated Fat: 8 g, Polyunsaturated Fat: 2 g), Cholesterol: 25 mg, Sodium: 400 mg, Fiber: 12 g, Sugars: 5 g

Glycemic Index: Lentils: Low (GI = 32), Feta cheese: Low (GI = 30), Cherry tomatoes: Low (GI = 15), Cucumber: Very Low (GI = 15), Red onion: Low (GI = 10)

28. Zucchini Noodle Salad with Pesto

Prep: 10 min | **Total:** 10 min | **Difficulty:** 1/5

Ingredients: Zucchini: 2 medium (400g, 14.1 oz), Cherry tomatoes, halved: 1 cup (150g, 5.29 oz), Fresh basil leaves: 1/2 cup (25g, 0.88 oz), Pine nuts: 2 tbsp (30g, 1.06 oz), Parmesan cheese, grated: 1/4 cup (25g, 0.88 oz), Olive oil: 2 tbsp (30 ml, 1.01 oz), Garlic: 1 clove (3g, 0.11 oz), Lemon juice: 1 tbsp (15 ml, 0.51 oz), Salt and pepper: to taste

1. **Preparation:** Spiralize the zucchini into noodles. Halve the cherry tomatoes. Mince the garlic.
2. **Pesto:** In a food processor, combine basil leaves, pine nuts, Parmesan cheese, olive oil, minced garlic, lemon juice, salt, and pepper. Blend until smooth.
3. **Mixing:** In a large bowl, combine zucchini noodles and cherry tomatoes. Add the pesto and toss gently to coat.
4. **Serving:** Serve immediately, garnished with extra pine nuts and basil leaves if desired.

Chef's Tips: *"For added protein, mix in some grilled chicken or shrimp. You can also add a handful of baby spinach or arugula for extra greens and nutrients."*

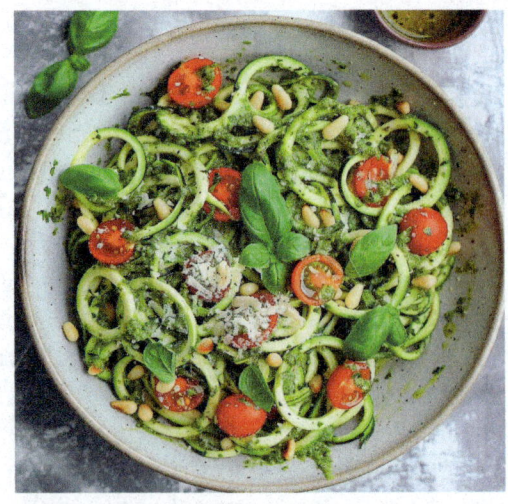

Nutritional Values: Calories: 250 kcal, Carbs: 14 g, Protein: 7 g, Fat: 20 g (Saturated Fat: 3 g, Monounsaturated Fat: 12 g, Polyunsaturated Fat: 2 g), Cholesterol: 5 mg, Sodium: 150 mg, Fiber: 4 g, Sugars: 5 g

Glycemic Index: Zucchini: Very Low (GI = 15), Cherry tomatoes: Low (GI = 15), Basil: Very Low (GI = 5), Pine nuts: Very Low (GI = 15), Parmesan cheese: Low (GI = 30)

LUNCH
Wrap It Up

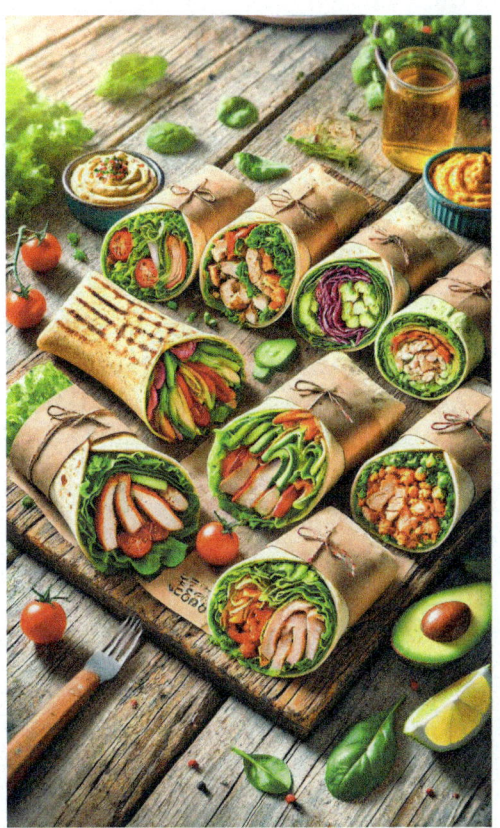

Note: These recipes are designed for one serving. To accommodate more people, simply multiply the ingredients by the desired number of servings.

The words "tablespoon" and "teaspoon" have been shortened to "tbsp" and "tsp".

29. Turkey and Avocado Wrap with Spinach

Prep: 10 min | **Total:** 10 min | **Difficulty:** 1/5

Ingredients: Whole wheat tortilla: 1 large (60g, 2.12 oz), Sliced turkey breast: 100g (3.53 oz), Fresh spinach: 1 cup (30g, 1.06 oz), Avocado: 1/2 medium (75g, 2.65 oz), Tomato, sliced: 1/2 medium (60g, 2.12 oz), Olive oil: 1 tsp (5 ml), Lemon juice: 1 tsp (5 ml), Salt and pepper: to taste

1. Preparation: Slice the avocado and tomato.
2. Assembly: Lay the tortilla flat and spread the olive oil and lemon juice evenly over it. Layer with spinach, sliced turkey, avocado, and tomato.
3. Flavoring: Season with salt and pepper.
4. Serving: Roll the tortilla tightly and cut in half. Serve immediately.

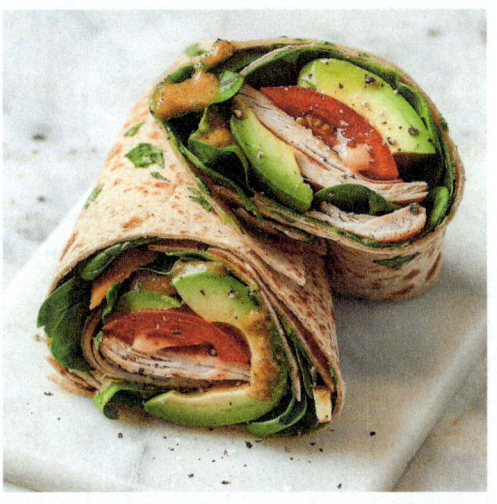

Nutritional Values: Calories: 350 kcal, Carbs: 30 g, Protein: 20 g, Fat: 18 g (Saturated Fat: 3 g, Monounsaturated Fat: 10 g, Polyunsaturated Fat: 2 g), Cholesterol: 45 mg, Sodium: 500 mg, Fiber: 8 g, Sugars: 2 g

Glycemic Index: Whole wheat tortilla: Medium (GI = 50), Sliced turkey breast: Low (GI = 0), Spinach: Very Low (GI = 15), Avocado: Very Low (GI = 15), Tomato: Low (GI = 15)

Chef's Tips: *"For extra crunch, add some thinly sliced cucumber or bell pepper."*

30. Grilled Chicken Caesar Wrap

Prep: 10 min | **Cook:** 10 min | **Total:** 20 min | **Difficulty:** 2/5

Ingredients: Whole wheat tortilla: 1 large (60g, 2.12 oz), Grilled chicken breast, sliced: 100g (3.53 oz), Romaine lettuce: 1 cup (50g, 1.76 oz), Parmesan cheese, grated: 2 tbsp (10g, 0.35 oz), Cherry tomatoes, halved: 1/2 cup (75g, 2.65 oz), Caesar dressing (low-fat): 2 tbsp (30 ml, 1.01 oz), Salt and pepper: to taste

1. **Preparation:** Grill the chicken breast if not pre-cooked, then slice it. Halve the cherry tomatoes.
2. **Assembly:** Lay the tortilla flat. Layer with romaine lettuce, grilled chicken, cherry tomatoes, and Parmesan cheese.
3. **Flavoring:** Drizzle Caesar dressing over the ingredients. Season with salt and pepper.
4. **Serving:** Roll the tortilla tightly and cut in half. Serve immediately.

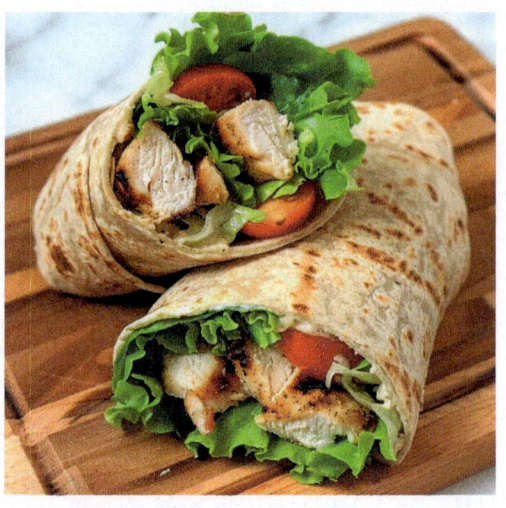

Nutritional Values: Calories: 370 kcal, Carbs: 30 g, Protein: 25 g, Fat: 18 g (Saturated Fat: 4 g, Monounsaturated Fat: 8 g, Polyunsaturated Fat: 2 g), Cholesterol: 55 mg, Sodium: 600 mg, Fiber: 6 g, Sugars: 2 g

Glycemic Index: Whole wheat tortilla: Medium (GI = 50), Grilled chicken breast: Low (GI = 0), Romaine lettuce: Very Low (GI = 5), Cherry tomatoes: Low (GI = 15), Parmesan cheese: Low (GI = 30)

Chef's Tips: *"For added flavor, include a few anchovy filets or a sprinkle of croutons."*

31. Black Bean and Corn Salsa Wrap

Prep: 10 min | **Total:** 10 min | **Difficulty:** 1/5

Ingredients: Whole wheat tortilla: 1 large (60g, 2.12 oz), Black beans, cooked: 1/2 cup (130g, 4.59 oz), Corn kernels: 1/2 cup (75g, 2.65 oz), Red bell pepper, diced: 1/2 cup (75g, 2.65 oz), Red onion, finely chopped: 1/4 cup (37.5g, 1.32 oz), Fresh cilantro, chopped: 2 tbsp (8g, 0.28 oz), Lime juice: 1 tbsp (15 ml, 0.51 oz), Olive oil: 1 tbsp (15 ml, 0.51 oz), Salt and pepper: to taste

1. **Preparation:** Rinse and drain black beans if using canned food. Dice the red bell pepper and finely chop the red onion.
2. **Mixing:** In a bowl, combine black beans, corn kernels, red bell pepper, red onion, and cilantro. Drizzle with lime juice and olive oil, then season with salt and pepper. Toss to mix well.
3. **Assembly:** Lay the tortilla flat and spread the black bean and corn salsa mixture evenly over it.
4. **Serving:** Roll the tortilla tightly and cut in half. Serve immediately.

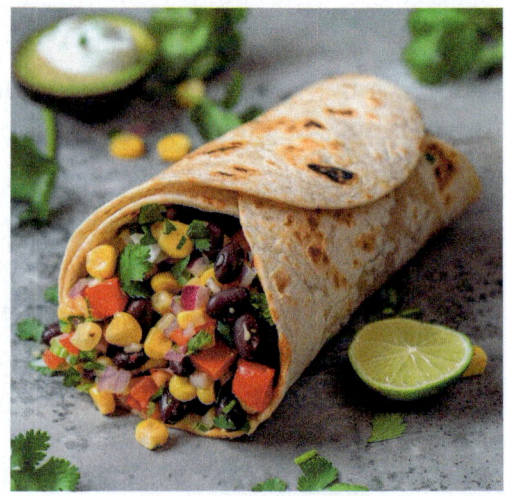

Nutritional Values: Calories: 340 kcal, Carbs: 55 g, Protein: 12 g, Fat: 10 g (Saturated Fat: 1.5 g, Monounsaturated Fat: 6 g, Polyunsaturated Fat: 2 g), Cholesterol: 0 mg, Sodium: 400 mg, Fiber: 12 g, Sugars: 8 g

Glycemic Index: Whole wheat tortilla: Medium (GI = 50), Black beans: Low (GI=30), Corn kernels: Medium (GI=60), Red bell pepper: Low (GI = 15), Red onion: Low (GI = 10)

Chef's Tips: *"For added creaminess, add a few slices of avocado or a dollop of Greek yogurt."*

32. Smoked Salmon and Cream Cheese Wrap

Prep: 10 min | **Total:** 10 min | **Difficulty:** 1/5

Ingredients: Whole wheat tortilla: 1 large (60g, 2.12 oz), Smoked salmon: 100g (3.53 oz), Cream cheese: 2 tbsp (30g, 1.06 oz), Fresh spinach: 1 cup (30g, 1.06 oz), Cucumber, thinly sliced: 1/2 cup (60g, 2.12 oz), Red onion, thinly sliced: 1/4 cup (37.5g, 1.32 oz), Capers: 1 tbsp (15g, 0.53 oz), Lemon juice: 1 tsp (5 ml), Salt and pepper: to taste

1. **Preparation:** Thinly slice the cucumber and red onion.
2. **Assembly:** Lay the tortilla flat and spread cream cheese evenly over it. Layer with fresh spinach, smoked salmon, cucumber slices, red onion slices, and capers.
3. **Flavoring:** Drizzle with lemon juice and season with salt and pepper.
4. **Serving:** Roll the tortilla tightly and cut in half. Serve immediately.

Chef's Tips: *"For added flavor, include a few fresh dill sprigs or a sprinkle of chives."*

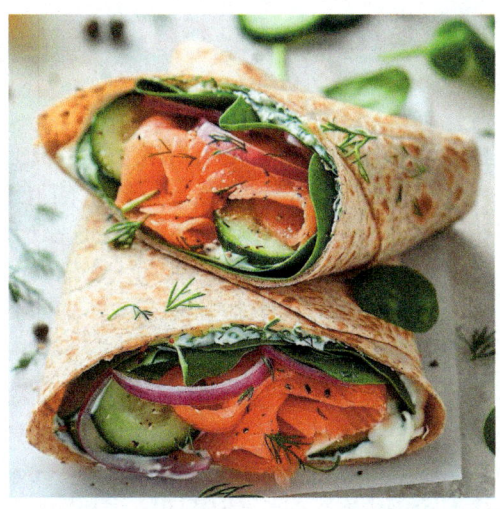

Nutritional Values: Calories: 330 kcal, Carbs: 30 g, Protein: 18 g, Fat: 18 g (Saturated Fat: 6 g, Monounsaturated Fat: 8 g, Polyunsaturated Fat: 2 g), Cholesterol: 40 mg, Sodium: 800 mg, Fiber: 6 g, Sugars: 3 g

Glycemic Index: Whole wheat tortilla: Medium (GI = 50), Smoked salmon: Low (GI = 0), Cream cheese: Low (GI = 30), Spinach: Very Low (GI = 15), Cucumber: Very Low (GI = 15), Red onion: Low (GI = 10)

33. Falafel and Hummus Wrap with Cucumber

Prep: 10 min | **Cook:** 10 min | **Total:** 20 min | **Difficulty:** 2/5

Ingredients: Whole wheat tortilla: 1 large (60g, 2.12 oz), Falafel balls: 4 (120g, 4.23 oz), Hummus: 2 tbsp (30g, 1.06 oz), Cucumber, thinly sliced: 1/2 cup (60g, 2.12 oz), Red onion, thinly sliced: 1/4 cup (37.5g, 1.32 oz), Fresh spinach: 1 cup (30g, 1.06 oz), Lemon juice: 1 tsp (5 ml), Olive oil: 1 tsp (5 ml), Salt and pepper: to taste

1. **Preparation:** Thinly slice the cucumber and red onion.
2. **Cooking:** Heat the falafel balls according to package instructions or homemade recipes.
3. **Assembly:** Lay the tortilla flat and spread hummus evenly over it. Layer with fresh spinach, cucumber slices, red onion slices, and falafel balls.
4. **Flavoring:** Drizzle with lemon juice and olive oil, season with salt and pepper.
5. **Serving:** Roll the tortilla tightly and cut in half. Serve immediately.

Chef's Tips: *"For extra flavor, add some chopped fresh mint or parsley."*

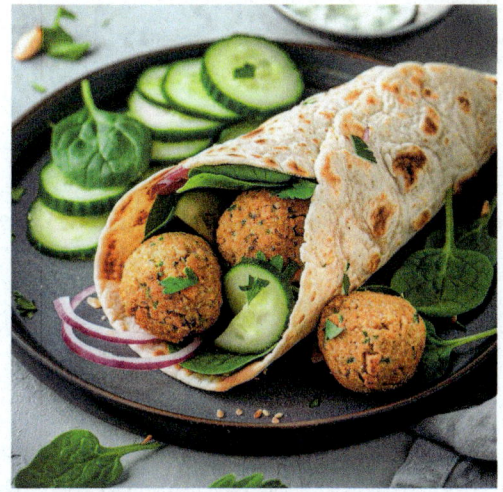

Nutritional Values: Calories: 380 kcal, Carbs: 45 g, Protein: 12 g, Fat: 16 g (Saturated Fat: 2 g, Monounsaturated Fat: 8 g, Polyunsaturated Fat: 4 g), Cholesterol: 0 mg, Sodium: 600 mg, Fiber: 10 g, Sugars: 2 g

Glycemic Index: Whole wheat tortilla: Medium (GI=50), Falafel: Medium (GI= 30-50), Hummus: Low (GI=15), Spinach: Very Low (GI= 15), Cucumber: Very Low (GI = 15), Red onion: Low (GI = 10)

34. Buffalo Chicken and Blue Cheese Wrap

Prep: 10 min | **Cook:** 10 min | **Total:** 20 min | **Difficulty:** 2/5

Ingredients: Whole wheat tortilla: 1 large (60g, 2.12 oz), Grilled chicken breast: 100g (3.53 oz), Buffalo sauce: 2 tbsp (30 ml, 1.01 oz), Blue cheese: 2 tbsp (30g, 1.06 oz), Lettuce: 1 cup (50g, 1.76 oz), Celery: 1/4 cup (30g, 1.06 oz), Olive oil: 1 tsp (5 ml), Salt and pepper: to taste

1. Preparation: Thinly slice the celery.
2. Cooking: Grill chicken if not pre-cooked, then slice and toss in buffalo sauce.
3. Assembly: Lay tortilla flat. Layer with lettuce, buffalo chicken, celery, and blue cheese.
4. Flavoring: Drizzle with olive oil and season to taste
5. Serving: Roll tortilla tightly and cut in half. Serve immediately.

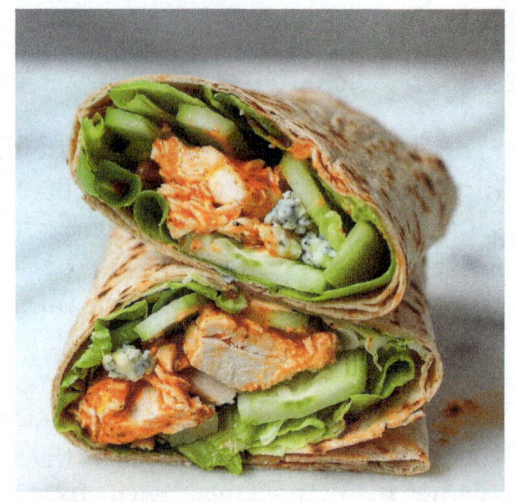

Nutritional Values: Calories: 380 kcal, Carbs: 30 g, Protein: 25 g, Fat: 20 g (Saturated Fat: 6 g, Monounsaturated Fat: 8 g, Polyunsaturated Fat: 2 g), Cholesterol: 70mg, Fiber: 6g, Sugars: 3g

Glycemic Index: Whole wheat tortilla: Medium (GI = 50), Grilled chicken breast: Low (GI = 0), Buffalo sauce: Medium (GI = 50), Blue cheese: Low (GI = 30), Lettuce: Very Low (GI = 5), Celery: Very Low (GI = 15)

Chef's Tips: *"For added crunch, include some chopped carrots or bell peppers."*

35. Mediterranean Veggie Wrap with Feta

Prep: 10 min | **Total:** 10 min | **Difficulty:** 1/5

Ingredients: Whole wheat tortilla: 1 large (60g, 2.12 oz), Feta cheese: 1/4 cup (60g, 2.12 oz), Hummus: 2 tbsp (30g, 1.06 oz), Cucumber: 1/2 cup (60g, 2.12 oz), Red bell pepper: 1/2 cup (75g, 2.65 oz), Kalamata olives: 1/4 cup (37.5g, 1.32 oz), Red onion: 1/4 cup (37.5g, 1.32 oz), Spinach: 1 cup (30g, 1.06 oz), Olive oil: 1 tsp (5 ml), Lemon juice: 1 tsp (5 ml), Salt and pepper: to taste

1. Preparation: Slice cucumber, red bell pepper, red onion, and olives.
2. Assembly: Lay the tortilla flat and spread hummus. Layer with spinach, cucumber, red bell pepper, olives, red onion, and feta cheese.
3. Flavoring: Drizzle with olive oil and lemon juice. Season with salt and pepper.
4. Serving: Roll the tortilla tightly and cut in half. Serve immediately.

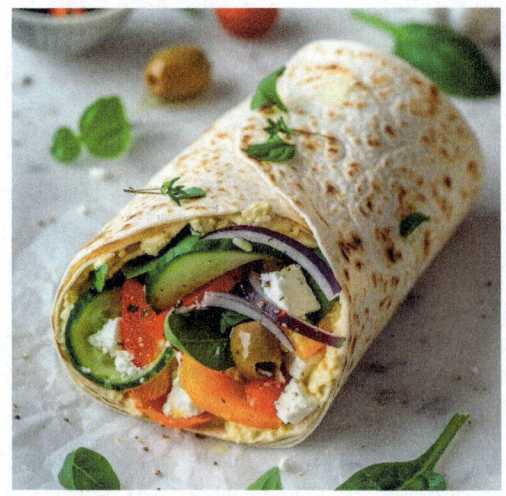

Nutritional Values: Calories: 350 kcal, Carbs: 35 g, Protein: 12 g, Fat: 18 g (Saturated Fat: 6 g, Monounsaturated Fat: 8 g, Polyunsaturated Fat: 2 g), Cholesterol: 25mg, Fiber: 8g, Sugars: 2 g

Glycemic Index: Whole wheat tortilla: Medium (GI = 50), Feta cheese: Low (GI = 30), Hummus: Low (GI = 15), Cucumber: Very Low (GI = 15), Red bell pepper: Low (GI = 15), Kalamata olives: Very Low (GI = 15), Red onion: Low (GI = 10), Spinach: Very Low (GI = 15)

Chef's Tips: *"For extra flavor, add some fresh basil or oregano leaves."*

LUNCH

Hearty Soups

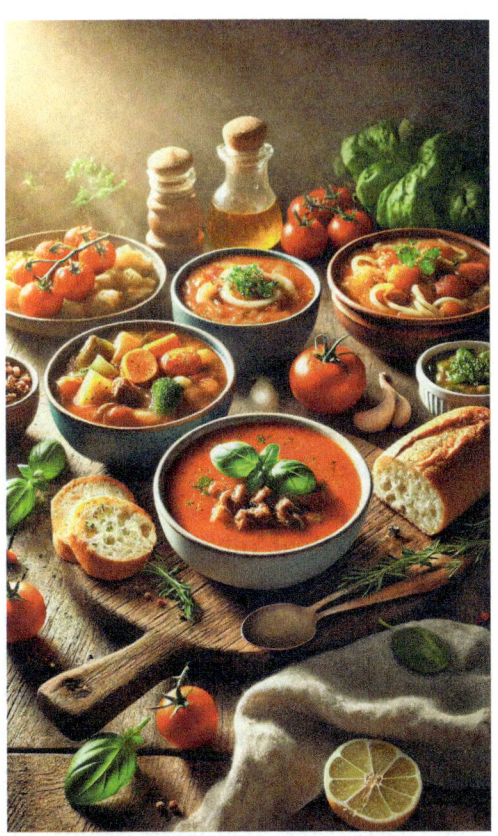

Note: These recipes are designed for one serving. To accommodate more people, simply multiply the ingredients by the desired number of servings.

The words "tablespoon" and "teaspoon" have been shortened to "tbsp" and "tsp".

36. Creamy Cauliflower and Leek Soup

Prep: 10 min | **Cook:** 25 min | **Total:** 35 min | **Difficulty:** 2/5

Ingredients: Cauliflower: 1 medium head (600g, 21.16 oz), Leeks, white and light green parts only: 2 (300g, 10.58 oz), Olive oil: 2 tbsp (30 ml, 1.01 oz), Garlic: 2 cloves (6g, 0.21 oz), Vegetable broth: 4 cups (960 ml), Unsweetened almond milk: 1 cup (240 ml), Salt and pepper: to taste, Fresh parsley, chopped: 2 tbsp (8g, 0.28 oz)

1. Preparation: Chop the cauliflower and leeks. Mince the garlic.
2. Cooking: Heat olive oil in a large pot over medium heat. Add leeks and garlic, sauté for 5 minutes. Add cauliflower and vegetable broth, bring to a boil. Reduce heat, cover, and simmer for 20 minutes until the cauliflower is tender.
3. Blending: Use an immersion blender to puree the soup until smooth. Stir in almond milk, season with salt and pepper.
4. Serving: Ladle into bowls and garnish with chopped parsley. Serve hot.

Chef's Tips: *"For added richness, stir in a tablespoon of Greek yogurt before serving."*

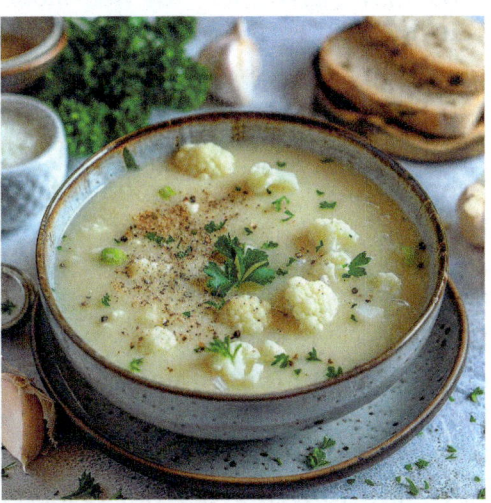

Nutritional Values: Calories: 150 kcal, Carbs: 18 g, Protein: 5 g, Fat: 8 g (Saturated Fat: 1 g, Monounsaturated Fat: 5 g, Polyunsaturated Fat: 1.5 g), Cholesterol: 0 mg, Sodium: 500 mg, Fiber: 6 g, Sugars: 6 g

Glycemic Index: Cauliflower: Very Low (GI = 15), Leeks: Low (GI = 15), Almond milk: Low (GI = 25)

41. Butternut Squash and Apple Soup

Prep: 10 min | **Cook:** 30 min | **Total:** 40 min | **Difficulty:** 2/5

Ingredients: Butternut squash, peeled and cubed: 4 cups (600g, 21.16 oz), Apple, peeled and chopped: 1 large (182g, 6.42 oz), Onion, diced: 1 medium (150g, 5.29 oz), Garlic, minced: 2 cloves (6g, 0.21 oz), Olive oil: 2 tbsp (30 ml, 1.01 oz), Vegetable broth: 4 cups (960 ml), Ground cinnamon: 1/2 tsp (1g, 0.04 oz), Ground nutmeg: 1/4 tsp (0.6g, 0.02 oz), Salt and pepper: to taste, Fresh thyme leaves: 1 tsp (1g, 0.04 oz)

1.Preparation: Peel and cube butternut squash, peel and chop apple, dice onion, and mince garlic.

2.Cooking: Heat olive oil in a large pot over medium heat. Sauté onion and garlic for 5 minutes. Add butternut squash, apple, and vegetable broth. Bring to a boil, then reduce heat and simmer for 25 minutes until squash and apple are tender.

3.Blending: Use an immersion blender to puree the soup until smooth. Stir in cinnamon, nutmeg, salt, and pepper.

4.Serving: Ladle into bowls and garnish with fresh thyme leaves. Serve hot.

Chef's Tips: *"For added creaminess, stir in a splash of coconut milk before serving."*

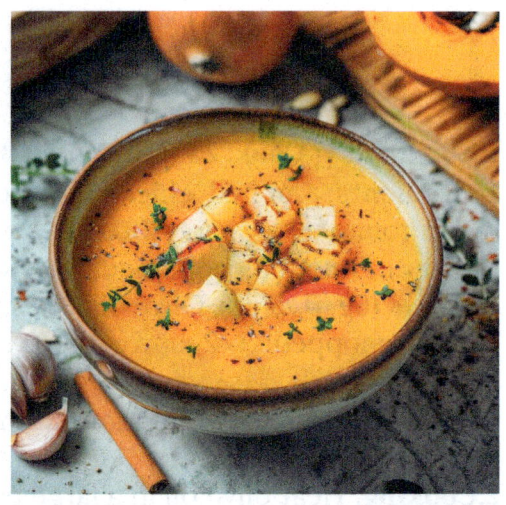

Nutritional Values: Calories: 180 kcal, Carbs: 35 g, Protein: 2 g, Fat: 5 g (Saturated Fat: 1 g, Monounsaturated Fat: 3 g, Polyunsaturated Fat: 1 g), Cholesterol: 0 mg, Sodium: 500 mg, Fiber: 7 g, Sugars: 10 g

Glycemic Index: Butternut squash: Medium (GI = 51), Apple: Medium (GI = 39), Onion: Low (GI = 10)

42. Zucchini and Fresh Herb Soup

Prep: 10 min | **Cook:** 20 min | **Total:** 30 min | **Difficulty:** 2/5

Ingredients: Zucchini, sliced: 4 cups (600g, 21.16 oz), Onion, diced: 1 medium (150g, 5.29 oz), Garlic, minced: 2 cloves (6g, 0.21 oz), Olive oil: 2 tbsp (30 ml, 1.01 oz), Vegetable broth: 4 cups (960 ml), Fresh parsley, chopped: 1/4 cup (15g, 0.53 oz), Fresh basil, chopped: 1/4 cup (15g, 0.53 oz), Salt and pepper: to taste, Lemon juice: 1 tbsp (15 ml)

1.Preparation: Slice zucchini, dice onion, and minced garlic. Chop fresh parsley and basil.

2.Cooking: Heat olive oil in a large pot over medium heat. Sauté onion and garlic for 5 minutes. Add zucchini and vegetable broth. Bring to a boil, then reduce heat and simmer for 15 minutes until zucchini is tender.

3.Blending: Use an immersion blender to puree the soup until smooth. Stir in fresh parsley, basil, salt, and pepper.

4.Serving: Ladle into bowls, drizzle with lemon juice, and serve hot.

Chef's Tips: *"For added richness, stir in a dollop of Greek yogurt or a splash of coconut milk before serving."*

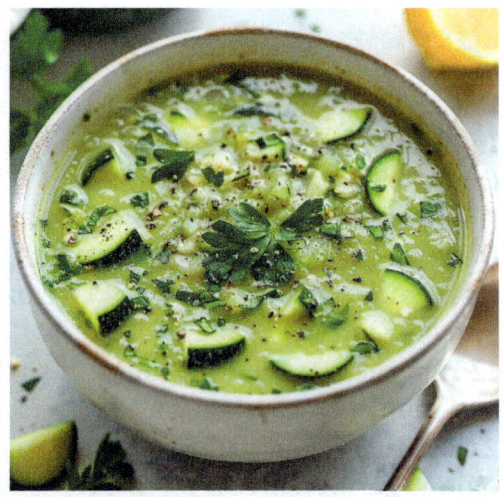

Nutritional Values: Calories: 150 kcal, Carbs: 20 g, Protein: 3 g, Fat: 7 g (Saturated Fat: 1 g, Monounsaturated Fat: 4 g, Polyunsaturated Fat: 1 g), Cholesterol: 0 mg, Sodium: 500 mg, Fiber: 5 g, Sugars: 6 g

Glycemic Index: Zucchini: Very Low (GI = 15), Onion: Low (GI = 10), Parsley: Very Low (GI = 5), Basil: Very Low (GI = 5)

DINNER
Vegetarian Ventures

Note: These recipes are designed for one serving. To accommodate more people, simply multiply the ingredients by the desired number of servings.

The words "tablespoon" and "teaspoon" have been shortened to "tbsp" and "tsp".

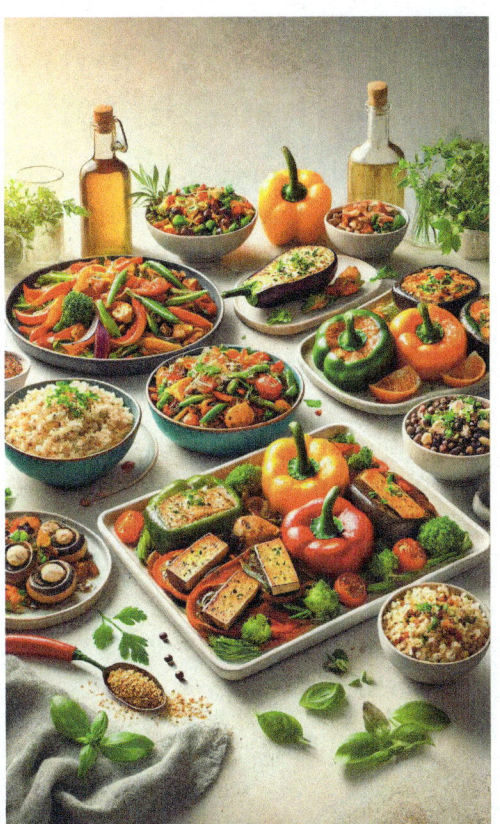

43. Stuffed Bell Peppers with Quinoa and Black Beans

Prep: 15 min | **Cook:** 30 min | **Total:** 45 min | **Difficulty:** 3/5
Ingredients: Bell peppers: 4 (600g, 21.16 oz), Quinoa: 1 cup (170g, 6 oz), Black beans: 1 cup (260g, 9.17 oz), Corn: 1/2 cup (75g, 2.65 oz), Diced tomatoes: 1 can (400g, 14.1 oz), Onion: 1 medium (150g, 5.29 oz), Garlic: 2 cloves (6g, 0.21 oz), Olive oil: 2 tbsp (30 ml, 1.01 oz), Cumin: 1 tsp (2g, 0.07 oz), Chili powder: 1 tsp (2g, 0.07 oz), Salt and pepper: to taste, Cilantro: 2 tbsp (8g, 0.28 oz), Cheese (optional): 1/2 cup (60g, 2.12 oz)
1. Preparation: Preheat the oven to 375°F (190°C). Halve and seed bell peppers. Dice onion and minced garlic.
2. Cooking: Cook quinoa. Sauté onion and garlic in olive oil for 5 min. Add black beans, corn, tomatoes, cumin, chili powder, salt, and pepper. Stir in quinoa.
3. Assembly: Stuff peppers with quinoa mixture. Place in a baking dish.
4. Baking: Cover with foil and bake for 25 min. Remove foil, add cheese if using, bake 5 more min.
5. Serving: Garnish with cilantro and serve hot.

Chef's Tips: *"For extra flavor, add a squeeze of lime juice before serving."*

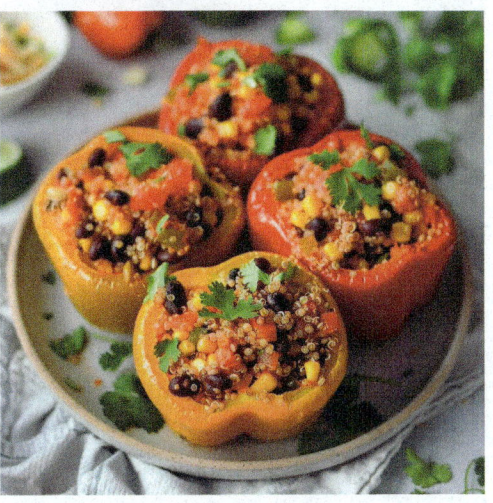

Nutritional Values: Calories: 250 kcal, Carbs: 45 g, Protein: 10 g, Fat: 7 g (Saturated Fat: 1 g, Monounsaturated Fat: 4 g, Polyunsaturated Fat: 1.5 g), Cholesterol: 0 mg, Sodium: 500 mg, Fiber: 12 g, Sugars: 10 g

Glycemic Index: Quinoa: Low (GI = 53), Black beans: Low (GI = 30), Corn: Medium (GI = 60), Bell peppers: Low (GI = 15), Onion: Low (GI = 10)

44. Eggplant Parmesan with Spinach and Ricotta

Prep: 15 min | **Cook:** 45 min | **Total:** 60 min | **Difficulty:** 3/5

Ingredients: Eggplant: 2 large (600g, 21.16 oz), Spinach: 2 cups (60g, 2.12 oz), Ricotta cheese: 1 cup (250g, 8.82 oz), Parmesan cheese: 1/2 cup (50g, 1.76 oz), Marinara sauce: 2 cups (480g, 16.93 oz), Olive oil: 2 tbsp (30 ml, 1.01 oz), Garlic powder: 1 tsp (2g, 0.07 oz), Salt and pepper: to taste, Basil: 2 tbsp (8g, 0.28 oz)

1. **Preparation:** Preheat the oven to 375°F (190°C). Slice eggplant. Rinse and chop spinach.
2. **Cooking:** Brush eggplant with olive oil, season with garlic powder, salt, and pepper. Bake for 20 min.
3. **Assembly:** Layer marinara sauce, eggplant, spinach, and ricotta in a baking dish. Repeat, top with Parmesan.
4. **Baking:** Cover with foil, bake for 20 min. Remove foil, bake 10 more min.
5. **Serving:** Garnish with basil and serve hot.

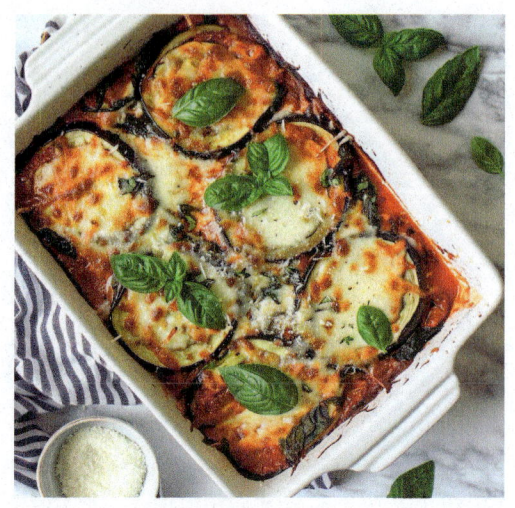

Nutritional Values: Calories: 300 kcal, Carbs: 25 g, Protein: 12 g, Fat: 18 g (Saturated Fat: 6 g, Monounsaturated Fat: 8 g, Polyunsaturated Fat: 2 g), Cholesterol: 30 mg, Sodium: 600 mg, Fiber: 8 g, Sugars: 7 g

Glycemic Index: Eggplant: Very Low (GI = 15), Spinach: Very Low (GI = 15), Ricotta cheese: Low (GI = 30), Parmesan cheese: Low (GI = 30), Marinara sauce: Low (GI = 30)

Chef's Tips: *"For extra flavor, add a layer of sautéed mushrooms or zucchini slices."*

45. Vegetable Stir-Fry with Tofu and Broccoli

Prep: 10 min | **Cook:** 15 min | **Total:** 25 min | **Difficulty:** 2/5

Ingredients: Tofu: 200g (7.05 oz), Broccoli: 2 cups (150g, 5.29 oz), Red bell pepper: 1 cup (150g, 5.29 oz), Carrot: 1 cup (130g, 4.59 oz), Snow peas: 1 cup (100g, 3.53 oz), Green onions: 1/4 cup (30g, 1.06 oz), Garlic: 2 cloves (6g, 0.21 oz), Soy sauce: 2 tbsp (30 ml, 1.01 oz), Olive oil: 2 tbsp (30 ml, 1.01 oz), Sesame seeds: 1 tbsp (15g, 0.53 oz), Cilantro: 2 tbsp (8g, 0.28 oz), Salt and pepper: to taste

1. **Preparation:** Cube tofu, cut broccoli, slice bell pepper, julienne carrot, chop green onions, mince garlic.
2. **Cooking:** Heat olive oil in a skillet over medium-high heat. Cook tofu until golden, 5-7 min. Remove tofu.
3. **Stir-Fry:** In the same skillet, add garlic and cook for 1 min. Add broccoli, bell pepper, carrot, and snow peas. Stir-fry 5-7 min.
4. **Mixing:** Return tofu, add soy sauce and green onions. Toss to combine.
5. **Serving:** Garnish with sesame seeds and cilantro. Serve hot.

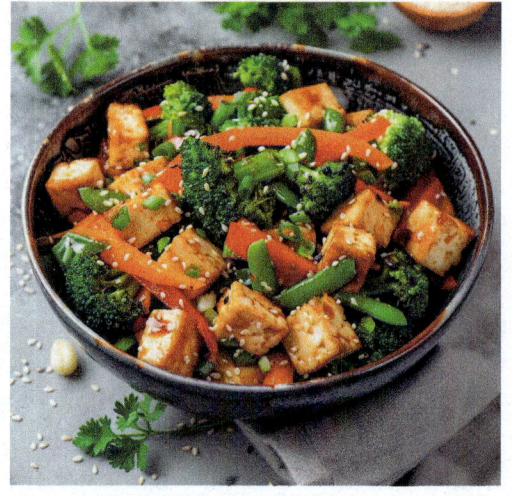

Nutritional Values: Calories: 250 kcal, Carbs: 20 g, Protein: 12 g, Fat: 15 g (Saturated Fat: 2 g, Monounsaturated Fat: 8 g, Polyunsaturated Fat: 4 g), Cholesterol: 0 mg, Sodium: 500 mg, Fiber: 6 g, Sugars: 6 g

Glycemic Index: Tofu: Low (GI = 15), Broccoli: Very Low (GI = 10), Red bell pepper: Low (GI = 15), Carrot: Low (GI = 35), Snow peas: Low (GI = 30)

Chef's Tips: *"For added flavor, drizzle with a bit of sesame oil before serving."*

46. Butternut Squash and Lentil Stew

Prep: 10 min | **Cook:** 30 min | **Total:** 40 min | **Difficulty:** 2/5

Ingredients: Butternut squash: 4 cups (600g, 21.16 oz), Lentils: 1 cup (200g, 7.05 oz), Onion: 1 medium (150g, 5.29 oz), Carrots: 1 cup (130g, 4.59 oz), Celery: 1 cup (100g, 3.53 oz), Garlic: 2 cloves (6g, 0.21 oz), Olive oil: 2 tbsp (30 ml, 1.01 oz), Vegetable broth: 6 cups (1440 ml), Cumin: 1 tsp (2g, 0.07 oz), Coriander: 1 tsp (2g, 0.07 oz), Turmeric: 1/2 tsp (1g, 0.04 oz), Salt and pepper: to taste, Cilantro: 2 tbsp (8g, 0.28 oz)

1. **Preparation:** Dice onion, carrots, celery, minced garlic, cube butternut squash.
2. **Cooking:** Heat olive oil in a pot. Sauté onion, garlic, carrots, and celery for 5 min. Add butternut squash, lentils, broth, cumin, coriander, and turmeric. Boil, reduce heat, simmer for 25-30 min.
3. **Seasoning:** Season with salt and pepper.
4. **Serving:** Garnish with cilantro. Serve hot.

Chef's Tips: *"For added richness, stir in a spoonful of Greek yogurt before serving."*

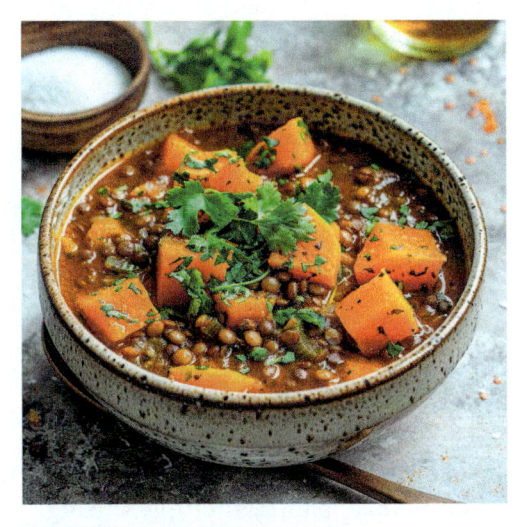

Nutritional Values: Calories: 250 kcal, Carbs: 45 g, Protein: 10 g, Fat: 6 g (Saturated Fat: 1 g, Monounsaturated Fat: 4 g, Polyunsaturated Fat: 1 g), Cholesterol: 0 mg, Sodium: 600 mg, Fiber: 15 g, Sugars: 12 g

Glycemic Index: Butternut squash: Medium (GI = 51), Lentils: Low (GI = 32), Carrots: Low (GI = 35), Celery: Very Low (GI = 15), Onion: Low (GI = 10)

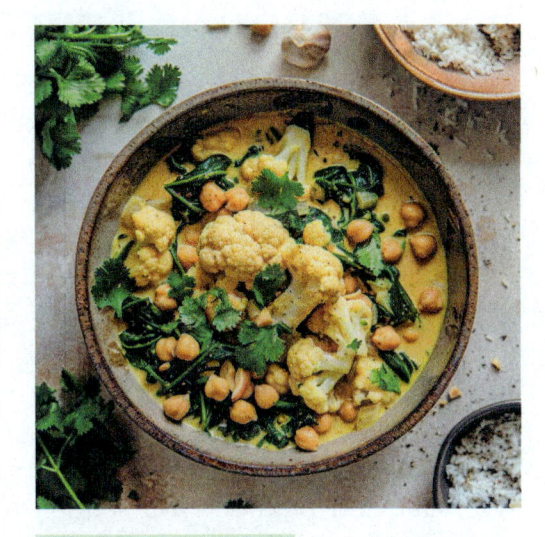

47. Cauliflower Curry with Chickpeas and Spinach

Prep: 10 min | **Cook:** 25 min | **Total:** 35 min | **Difficulty:** 2/5

Ingredients: Cauliflower: 4 cups (600g, 21.16 oz), Chickpeas: 1 can (400g, 14.1 oz), Spinach: 2 cups (60g, 2.12 oz), Onion: 1 medium (150g, 5.29 oz), Garlic: 2 cloves (6g, 0.21 oz), Ginger: 1 tbsp (6g, 0.21 oz), Olive oil: 2 tbsp (30 ml, 1.01 oz), Coconut milk: 1 cup (240 ml), Vegetable broth: 1 cup (240 ml), Curry powder: 1 tbsp (6g, 0.21 oz), Cumin: 1 tsp (2g, 0.07 oz), Turmeric: 1 tsp (2g, 0.07 oz), Salt and pepper: to taste, Cilantro: 2 tbsp (8g, 0.28 oz)

1. **Preparation:** Dice onion, mince garlic and ginger, chop cauliflower into florets.
2. **Cooking:** Heat olive oil in a pot. Sauté onion, garlic, and ginger for 5 min. Add cauliflower, curry powder, cumin, turmeric and cook for 3 min.
3. **Simmering:** Add chickpeas, coconut milk, and broth. Boil, reduce heat, simmer 15 min until cauliflower is tender.
4. **Mixing:** Stir in spinach, cook for 2 min. Season with salt and pepper.
5. **Serving:** Garnish with cilantro. Serve hot.

Chef's Tips: *"For added texture, top with toasted cashews or almonds."*

Nutritional Values: Calories: 270 kcal, Carbs: 30 g, Protein: 10 g, Fat: 14 g (Saturated Fat: 7 g, Monounsaturated Fat: 4 g, Polyunsaturated Fat: 1 g), Cholesterol: 0 mg, Sodium: 600 mg, Fiber: 10 g, Sugars: 7 g

Glycemic Index: Cauliflower: Very Low (GI = 15), Chickpeas: Low (GI = 28), Spinach: Very Low (GI = 15), Coconut milk: Low (GI = 41), Onion: Low (GI = 10)

DINNER
Seafood Selections

Note: These recipes are designed for one serving. To accommodate more people, simply multiply the ingredients by the desired number of servings.

The words "tablespoon" and "teaspoon" have been shortened to "tbsp" and "tsp".

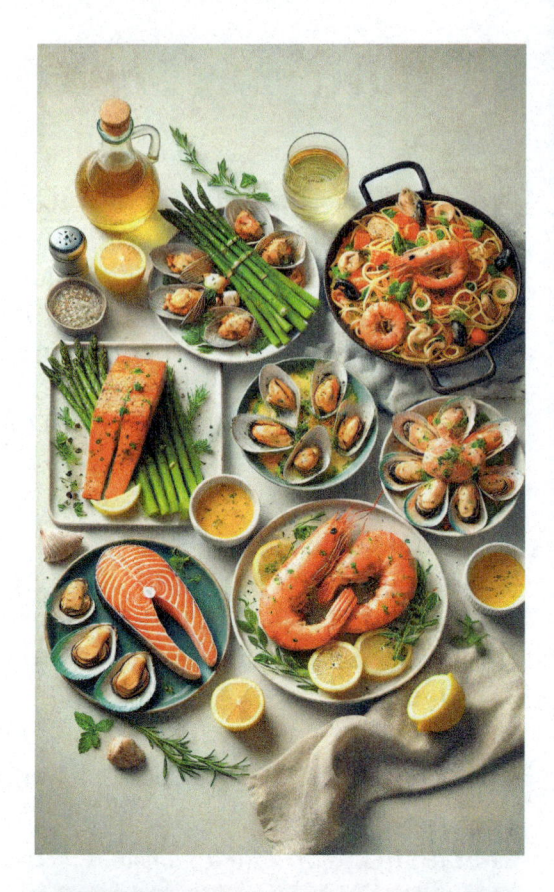

48. Grilled Salmon with Asparagus and Lemon-Dill Sauce

Prep: 10 min | **Cook:** 15 min | **Total:** 25 min | **Difficulty:** 2/5
Ingredients: Salmon fillets: 2 (300g, 10.58 oz), Asparagus, trimmed: 1 bunch (250g, 8.82 oz), Olive oil: 2 tbsp (30 ml, 1.01 oz), Salt and pepper: to taste
Lemon-Dill Sauce: Greek yogurt: 1/2 cup (120g, 4.23 oz), Fresh dill, chopped: 2 tbsp (8g, 0.28 oz), Lemon juice: 2 tbsp (30 ml, 1.01 oz), Lemon zest: 1 tsp (2g, 0.07 oz), Garlic, minced: 1 clove (3g, 0.11 oz), Salt and pepper: to taste
1. Preparation: Preheat grill to medium-high heat. Trim asparagus. Mix all sauce ingredients in a bowl.
2. Cooking: Brush salmon and asparagus with olive oil, season with salt and pepper. Grill salmon for 4-5 min. per side until cooked through. Grill asparagus for 5-7 min. until tender.
3. Assembly: Place grilled salmon and asparagus on plates.
4. Serving: Drizzle lemon-dill sauce over salmon. Serve immediately.

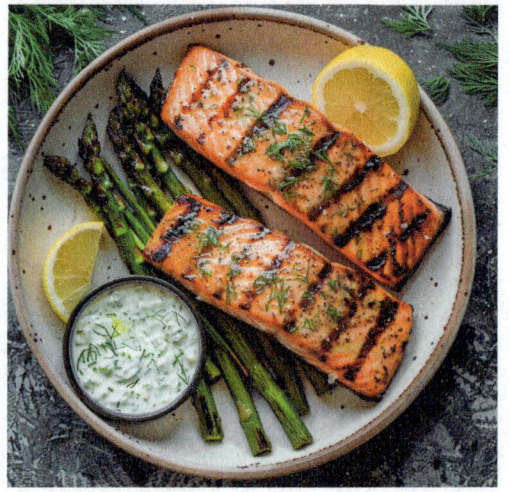

Nutritional Values: Calories: 350 kcal, Carbs: 10 g, Protein: 35 g, Fat: 20 g (Saturated Fat: 3 g, Monounsaturated Fat: 10 g, Polyunsaturated Fat: 5 g), Cholesterol: 80 mg, Sodium: 300 mg, Fiber: 4 g, Sugars: 4 g

Glycemic Index: Salmon: Low (GI = 0), Asparagus: Very Low (GI = 15), Greek yogurt: Low (GI = 30)

Chef's Tips: *"For extra flavor, marinate the salmon in olive oil, lemon juice, and dill for 30 minutes before grilling."*

49. Shrimp and Quinoa Paella

Prep: 10 min | **Cook:** 30 min | **Total:** 40 min | **Difficulty:** 3/5

Ingredients: Shrimp, peeled and deveined: 300g (10.58 oz), Quinoa: 1 cup (170g, 6 oz), Olive oil: 2 tbsp (30 ml, 1.01 oz), Onion, diced: 1 medium (150g, 5.29 oz), Red bell pepper, diced: 1 cup (150g, 5.29 oz), Green peas: 1 cup (150g, 5.29 oz), Garlic, minced: 2 cloves (6g, 0.21 oz), Tomato paste: 2 tbsp (30g, 1.06 oz), Saffron threads: a pinch, Chicken or vegetable broth: 3 cups (720 ml), Paprika: 1 tsp (2g, 0.07 oz), Salt and pepper: to taste, Fresh parsley, chopped: 2 tbsp (8g, 0.28 oz), Lemon wedges: for serving

1. Preparation: Dice onion and red bell pepper. Mince garlic. Rinse quinoa.

2. Cooking: Heat olive oil in a large pan over medium heat. Sauté onion, garlic, and red bell pepper for 5 min. Add quinoa, tomato paste, saffron, and paprika, cook for 2 min. Pour in broth, bring to a boil, then reduce heat and simmer for 15 min.

3. Adding Shrimp: Stir in shrimp and green peas, cook for another 5 minutes until shrimp are pink and quinoa is tender.

4. Serving: Season with salt and pepper. Garnish with fresh parsley and serve with lemon wedges.

Chef's Tips: *"For extra flavor, add a splash of white wine while cooking the quinoa."*

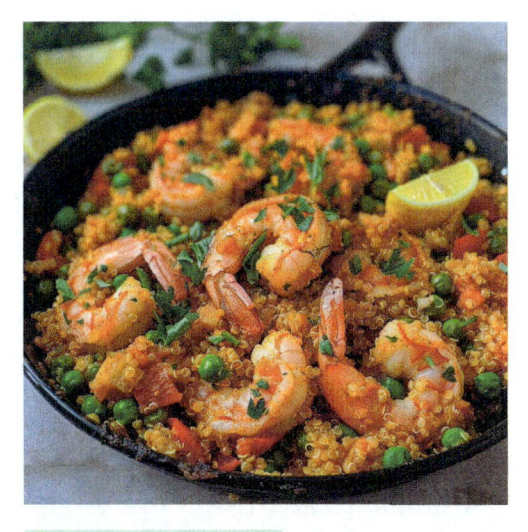

Nutritional Values: Calories: 350 kcal, Carbs: 35 g, Protein: 25 g, Fat: 12 g (Saturated Fat: 2 g, Monounsaturated Fat: 7 g, Polyunsaturated Fat: 2 g), Cholesterol: 150 mg, Sodium: 600 mg, Fiber: 6 g, Sugars: 6 g

Glycemic Index: Shrimp: Low (GI = 0), Quinoa: Low (GI = 53), Red bell pepper: Low (GI = 15), Green peas: Low (GI = 22), Onion: Low (GI = 10)

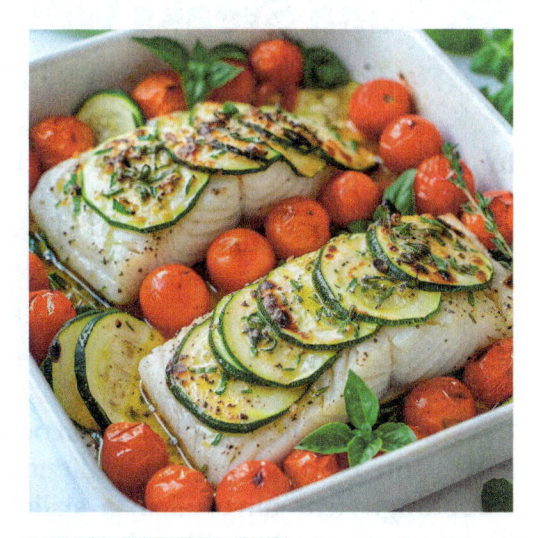

50. Baked Cod with Herbed Tomatoes and Zucchini

Prep: 10 min | **Cook:** 20 min | **Total:** 30 min | **Difficulty:** 2/5

Ingredients: Cod fillets: 2 (300g, 10.58 oz), Cherry tomatoes, halved: 1 cup (150g, 5.29 oz), Zucchini, sliced: 1 medium (200g, 7.05 oz), Olive oil: 2 tbsp (30 ml, 1.01 oz), Fresh basil, chopped: 2 tbsp (8g, 0.28 oz), Fresh thyme, chopped: 1 tbsp (4g, 0.14 oz), Garlic, minced: 2 cloves (6g, 0.21 oz), Lemon juice: 2 tbsp (30 ml, 1.01 oz), Salt and pepper: to taste

1. Preparation: Preheat the oven to 375°F (190°C). Halve cherry tomatoes, slice zucchini, mince garlic, and chop basil and thyme.

2. Assembly: Place cod fillets in a baking dish. Arrange cherry tomatoes and zucchini around the fish. Drizzle with olive oil and lemon juice. Sprinkle with garlic, basil, thyme, salt, and pepper.

3. Baking: Bake in a preheated oven for 20 minutes until the fish is opaque and flakes easily with a fork.

4. Serving: Serve hot with a garnish of fresh herbs.

Chef's Tips: *"For added flavor, marinate the cod in olive oil, lemon juice, and herbs for 30 minutes before baking."*

Nutritional Values: Calories: 250 kcal, Carbs: 10 g, Protein: 30 g, Fat: 12 g (Saturated Fat: 2 g, Monounsaturated Fat: 8 g, Polyunsaturated Fat: 2 g), Cholesterol: 70 mg, Sodium: 300 mg, Fiber: 3 g, Sugars: 7 g

Glycemic Index: Cod: Low (GI = 0), Cherry tomatoes: Low (GI = 15), Zucchini: Very Low (GI = 15)

54. Turkey Meatballs in Tomato Basil Sauce

Prep: 15 min | **Cook:** 25 min | **Total:** 40 min | **Difficulty: 3/5**

Ingredients: Ground turkey: 1 lb (450g), Breadcrumbs: 1/2 cup (60g), Egg: 1, Parmesan cheese (grated): 1/4 cup (30g), Garlic (minced): 2 cloves, Fresh basil (chopped): 2 tbsp (30ml), Salt: 1 tsp (5g), Black pepper: 1/2 tsp (2.5g), Olive oil: 1 tbsp (15ml), Onion (chopped): 1 medium (150g), Canned crushed tomatoes: 28 oz (800g), Dried oregano: 1 tsp (5g), Red pepper flakes: 1/4 tsp (1.25g)

1. **Preparation:** Mix ground turkey, breadcrumbs, egg, Parmesan, garlic, basil, salt, and pepper. Form into 1-inch meatballs.
2. **Cooking:** Preheat the oven to 375°F (190°C). Dice onion and minced garlic. Heat olive oil in a skillet, cook onion until translucent (5 minutes). Brown meatballs (8-10 minutes). Remove meatballs, add tomatoes, oregano, and red pepper flakes to skillet. Simmer, return meatballs, cook 15 minutes.
3. **Assembly:** Stir fresh basil into the sauce just before serving.
4. **Serving:** Serve meatballs with sauce over whole grain pasta or zucchini noodles, garnish with Parmesan and basil.

Chef's Tips: *"Add red wine to sauce for extra flavor. Include chopped spinach in meatballs for added nutrients".*

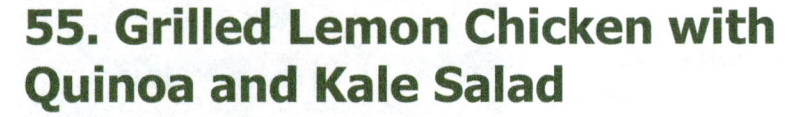

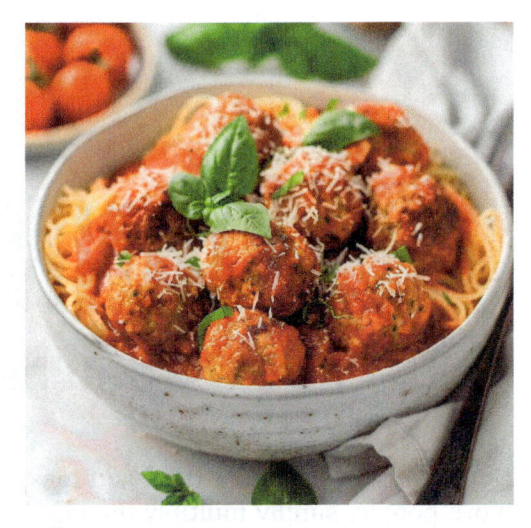

Nutritional Values: Calories: 350 kcal, Carbs: 20 g, Protein: 30 g, Fat: 18 g (Saturated Fat: 4 g, Monounsaturated Fat: 10 g, Polyunsaturated Fat: 2 g), Cholesterol: 100 mg, Sodium: 500 mg, Fiber: 5 g, Sugars: 6 g

Glycemic Index: Ground turkey: Low (GI = 0), Bread crumbs: Medium (GI = 65), Crushed tomatoes: Low (GI = 15), Onion: Low (GI = 10)

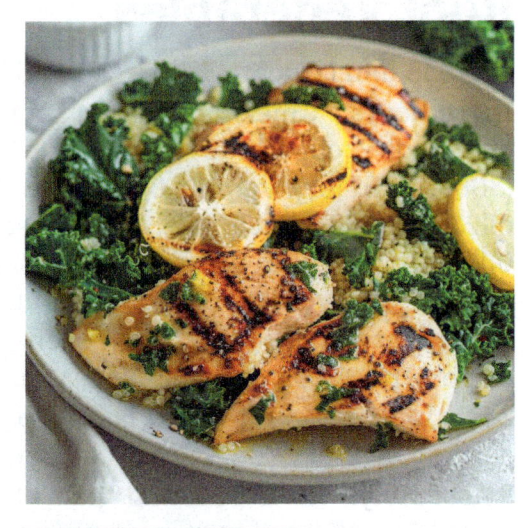

55. Grilled Lemon Chicken with Quinoa and Kale Salad

Prep: 10 min | **Cook:** 20 min | **Total:** 30 min | **Difficulty: 2/5**

Ingredients: Chicken breasts: 2 (300g, 10.58 oz), Quinoa: 1 cup (170g, 6 oz), Kale, chopped: 2 cups (60g, 2.12 oz), Olive oil: 3 tbsp (45 ml, 1.52 oz), Lemon juice: 2 tbsp (30 ml, 1.01 oz), Lemon zest: 1 tsp (2g, 0.07 oz), Garlic, minced: 2 cloves (6g, 0.21 oz), Salt and pepper: to taste

1. **Preparation:** Cook quinoa. Chop kale and mince garlic.
2. **Marinating:** Mix 2 tbsp olive oil, lemon juice, lemon zest, garlic, salt, and pepper. Marinate chicken breasts for 15 min.
3. **Grilling:** Grill chicken over medium heat, 6-7 min per side until cooked through.
4. **Salad:** Toss quinoa and kale with 1 tbsp olive oil, salt, and pepper.
5. **Serving:** Serve grilled chicken on top of quinoa and kale salad. Garnish with lemon slices.

Chef's Tips: *"Add feta cheese or toasted pine nuts to the salad for extra flavor."*

Nutritional Values: Calories: 400 kcal, Carbs: 35 g, Protein: 35 g, Fat: 15 g (Saturated Fat: 3 g, Monounsaturated Fat: 9 g, Polyunsaturated Fat: 2 g), Cholesterol: 80 mg, Sodium: 350 mg, Fiber: 6 g, Sugars: 2 g

Glycemic Index: Chicken breast: Low (GI = 0), Quinoa: Low (GI = 53), Kale: Very Low (GI = 15)

56. Beef Stir-Fry with Bell Peppers and Snow Peas

Prep: 10 min | **Cook:** 15 min | **Total:** 25 min | **Difficulty:** 2/5

Ingredients: Beef sirloin, thinly sliced: 300g (10.58 oz), Bell peppers, sliced: 2 cups (300g, 10.58 oz), Snow peas: 1 cup (100g, 3.53 oz), Garlic, minced: 2 cloves (6g, 0.21 oz), Soy sauce (low-sodium): 3 tbsp (45 ml, 1.52 oz), Olive oil: 2 tbsp (30 ml, 1.01 oz), Fresh ginger, grated: 1 tbsp (6g, 0.21 oz), Salt and pepper: to taste

1. **Preparation:** Thinly slice beef and bell peppers. Mince garlic and grate ginger.
2. **Cooking:** Heat olive oil in a skillet over medium-high heat. Sauté garlic and ginger for 1 minute until fragrant. Add beef and cook until browned, about 3-4 minutes.
3. **Stir-Fry:** Add bell peppers and snow peas to the skillet. Stir-fry for 5-7 minutes until vegetables are tender-crisp. Add soy sauce and cook for an additional 2 minutes.
4. **Serving:** Season with salt and pepper to taste. Serve hot.

Chef's Tips: *"For added flavor, sprinkle with sesame seeds or a dash of sesame oil before serving."*

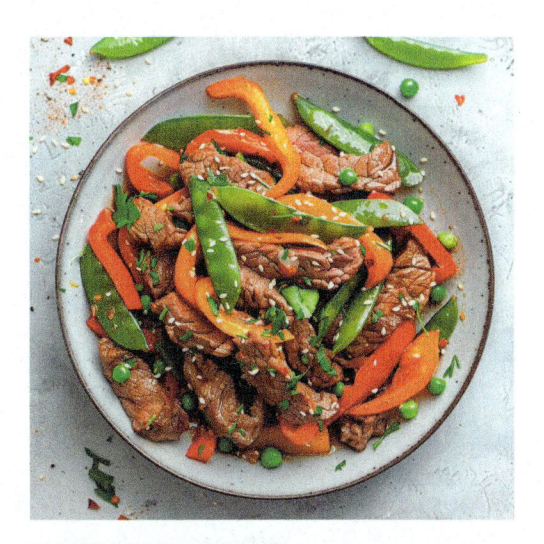

Nutritional Values: Calories: 350 kcal, Carbs: 15 g, Protein: 30 g, Fat: 18 g (Saturated Fat: 6 g, Monounsaturated Fat: 8 g, Polyunsaturated Fat: 2 g), Cholesterol: 70 mg, Sodium: 600 mg, Fiber: 5 g, Sugars: 6 g

Glycemic Index: Beef: Low (GI = 0), Bell peppers: Low (GI = 15), Snow peas: Low (GI = 30)

57. Pork Tenderloin with Apple and Sage

Prep: 10 min | **Cook:** 25 min | **Total:** 35 min | **Difficulty:** 3/5

Ingredients: Pork tenderloin: 500g (17.64 oz), Apples, sliced: 2 (300g, 10.58 oz), Fresh sage, chopped: 2 tbsp (8g, 0.28 oz), Olive oil: 2 tbsp (30 ml, 1.01 oz), Garlic, minced: 2 cloves (6g, 0.21 oz), Onion, sliced: 1 medium (150g, 5.29 oz), Chicken broth: 1/2 cup (120 ml), Salt and pepper: to taste

1. **Preparation:** Preheat the oven to 375°F (190°C). Slice apples and onion, mince garlic, and chop sage.
2. **Cooking:** Heat 1 tbsp olive oil in an oven-safe skillet over medium-high heat. Season pork tenderloin with salt and pepper. Sear pork on all sides until browned, about 4-5 min.
3. **Baking:** Add sliced apples, onion, garlic, and sage to the skillet. Pour in chicken broth. Transfer the skillet to the preheated oven and bake for 20-25 minutes until pork is cooked through.
4. **Serving:** Let the pork rest for 5 minutes before slicing. Serve with apples and onions.

Chef's Tips: *"For extra flavor, marinate the pork in olive oil, garlic, and sage for 1 hour before cooking."*

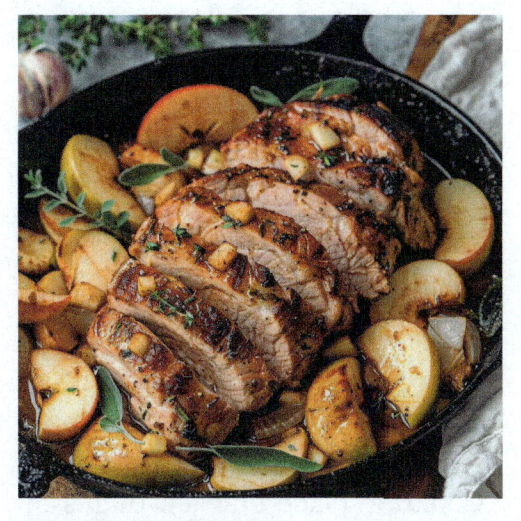

Nutritional Values: Calories: 350 kcal, Carbs: 20 g, Protein: 30 g, Fat: 15 g (Saturated Fat: 3 g, Monounsaturated Fat: 9 g, Polyunsaturated Fat: 2 g), Cholesterol: 80 mg, Sodium: 300 mg, Fiber: 4 g, Sugars: 13 g

Glycemic Index: Pork tenderloin: Low (GI = 0), Apples: Medium (GI = 39), Onion: Low (GI = 10)

58. Lamb Chops with Rosemary and Garlic

Prep: 10 min | **Cook:** 15 min | **Total:** 25 min | **Difficulty: 3/5**

Ingredients: Lamb chops: 4 (400g, 14.11 oz), Fresh rosemary, chopped: 2 tbsp (8g, 0.28 oz), Garlic, minced: 3 cloves (9g, 0.32 oz), Olive oil: 2 tbsp (30 ml, 1.01 oz), Salt and pepper: to taste, Lemon wedges: for serving

1. Preparation: Mince garlic and chop rosemary. Season lamb chops with salt, pepper, garlic, and rosemary.
2. Marinating: Drizzle with olive oil and let marinate for at least 15 minutes.
3. Cooking: Heat a skillet over medium-high heat. Sear lamb chops for 3-4 minutes per side for medium-rare, or until desired doneness.
4. Serving: Serve lamb chops with lemon wedges.

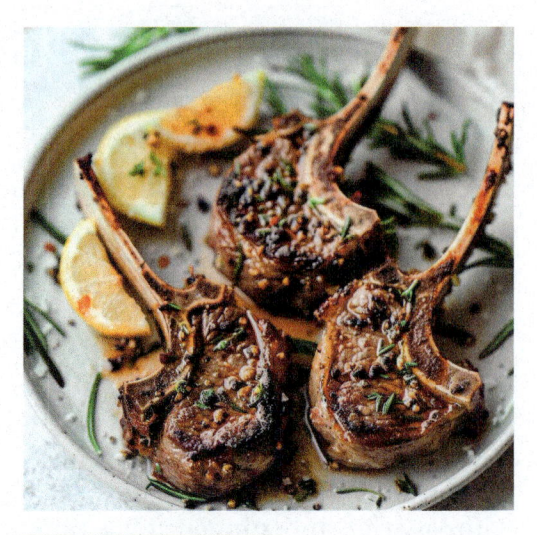

Nutritional Values: Calories: 420 kcal, Carbs: 2 g, Protein: 35 g, Fat: 30 g (Saturated Fat: 12 g, Monounsaturated Fat: 14 g, Polyunsaturated Fat: 2 g), Cholesterol: 110 mg, Sodium: 250 mg, Fiber: 0 g, Sugars: 1 g

Glycemic Index: Lamb chops: Low (GI = 0), Garlic: Low (GI = 10), Rosemary: Very Low (GI = 5)

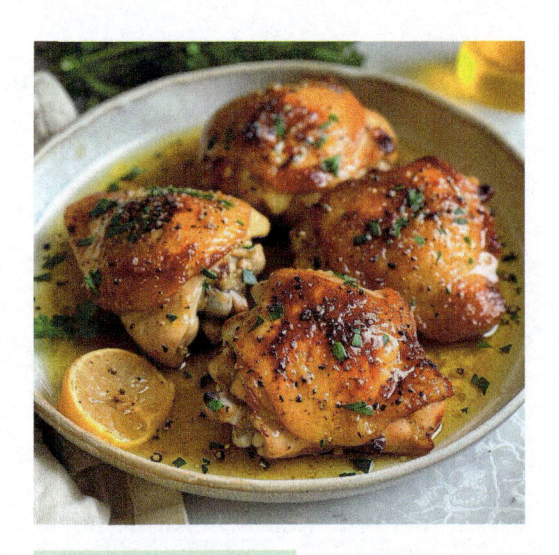

Chef's Tips: *"For extra flavor, add a splash of balsamic vinegar to the skillet while searing the lamb chops."*

59. Honey Mustard Glazed Chicken Thighs

Prep: 10 min | **Cook:** 25 min | **Total:** 35 min | **Difficulty: 2/5**

Ingredients: Chicken thighs: 4 (600g, 21.16 oz), Dijon mustard: 2 tbsp (30g, 1.06 oz), Stevia: 1 tsp (4g, 0.14 oz), Olive oil: 2 tbsp (30 ml, 1.01 oz), Garlic, minced: 2 cloves (6g, 0.21 oz), Salt and pepper: to taste, Fresh parsley, chopped: 2 tbsp (8g, 0.28 oz)

1. Preparation: Preheat the oven to 375°F (190°C). Mince garlic.
2. Marinating: In a bowl, mix Dijon mustard, stevia, olive oil, minced garlic, salt, and pepper. Coat chicken thighs with the mixture.
3. Cooking: Place chicken thighs in a baking dish and bake for 25 minutes until cooked through.
4. Serving: Garnish with fresh parsley and serve hot.

Nutritional Values: Calories: 300 kcal, Carbs: 2 g, Protein: 30 g, Fat: 18 g (Saturated Fat: 4 g, Monounsaturated Fat: 10 g, Polyunsaturated Fat: 2 g), Cholesterol: 90 mg, Sodium: 400 mg, Fiber: 0 g, Sugars: 2 g

Glycemic Index: Chicken thighs: Low (GI = 0), Dijon mustard: Low (GI = 10), Stevia: Very Low (GI = 0)

Chef's Tips: *"For added flavor, marinate the chicken for at least 1 hour before cooking."*

DINNER

Low-Carb Comforts

Note: These recipes are designed for one serving. To accommodate more people, simply multiply the ingredients by the desired number of servings.

The words "tablespoon" and "teaspoon" have been shortened to "tbsp" and "tsp".

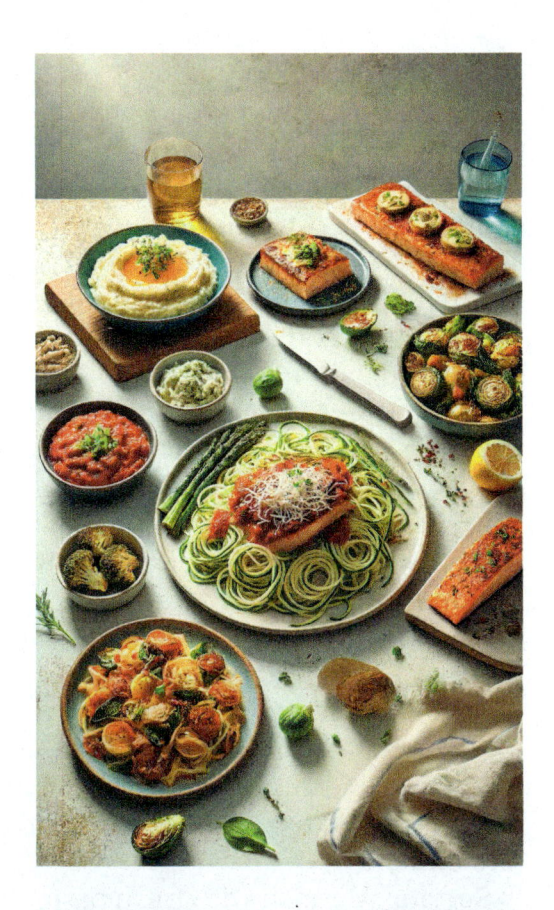

60. Spaghetti Squash Carbonara

Prep: 15 min | **Cook:** 25 min | **Total:** 40 min | **Difficulty: 2/5**

Ingredients: Spaghetti squash: 1 medium (800g, 28.22 oz), Bacon: 4 slices (120g, 4.23 oz), Eggs: 2 large, Parmesan cheese, grated: 1/2 cup (50g, 1.76 oz), Garlic, minced: 2 cloves (6g, 0.21 oz), Salt and pepper: to taste, Fresh parsley, chopped: 2 tbsp (8g, 0.28 oz)

1. Preparation: Preheat oven to 400°F (200°C). Halve spaghetti squash, scoop out seeds, and place cut side down on a baking sheet. Bake for 30-35 minutes until tender. Let cool slightly, then scrape flesh into strands.

2. Cooking: While the squash is baking, cook bacon in a skillet over medium heat until crispy. Remove bacon, crumble, and set aside. In the same skillet, add minced garlic and cook for 1 minute.

3. Assembly: In a bowl, whisk eggs and Parmesan cheese together. Add cooked spaghetti squash, crumbled bacon, and garlic. Toss to combine and cook over low heat until the sauce thickens slightly. Season with salt and pepper.

4. Serving: Garnish with fresh parsley. Serve immediately.

Chef's Tips: *"For added flavor, mix in some sautéed mushrooms or spinach before serving."*

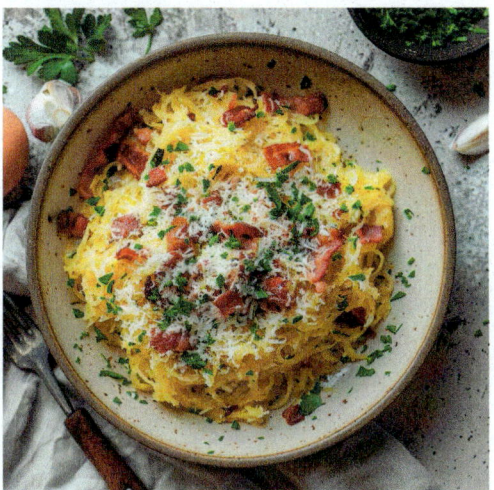

Nutritional Values: Calories: 204 kcal, Carbs: 8.75 g, Protein: 12.45 g, Fat: 14.83 g (Saturated Fat: 5.2 g, Monounsaturated Fat: 6.5 g, Polyunsaturated Fat: 1.2 g), Cholesterol: 103 mg, Sodium: 431 mg, Fiber: 1.73 g, Sugars: 2 g

Glycemic Index: Spaghetti Squash: Very Low (GI = 20), Eggs: Very Low (GI = 0), Parmesan Cheese: Very Low (GI = 0), Olive Oil: Very Low (GI = 0), Garlic: Low (GI = 30), Salt: Very Low (GI = 0), Pepper: Very Low (GI = 0), Parsley: Very Low (GI = 0)

61. Cauliflower Fried Rice with Chicken and Vegetables

Prep: 10 min | **Cook:** 15 min | **Total:** 25 min | **Difficulty:** 2/5

Ingredients: Cauliflower (riced): 1 medium head (600g), Mozzarella cheese (shredded): 1 cup (100g), Parmesan cheese (grated): 1/4 cup (25g), Egg: 1, Italian seasoning: 1 tsp (5g), Salt: 1/2 tsp (2.5g), Black pepper: 1/2 tsp (2.5g), Olive oil: 1 tbsp (15ml), Tomato sauce: 1/2 cup (120ml), Bell pepper (sliced): 1/2 cup (75g), Red onion (sliced): 1/4 cup (35g), Mushrooms (sliced): 1/2 cup (75g), Cherry tomatoes (halved): 1/2 cup (75g), Fresh basil (for garnish): 2 tbsp (30ml)

1. **Preparation:** Preheat oven to 400°F (200°C), line a baking sheet with parchment paper, steam riced cauliflower until tender, squeeze out moisture, mix cauliflower, mozzarella, Parmesan, egg, Italian seasoning, salt, and pepper.
2. **Crust Baking:** Form mixture into a crust on the baking sheet, bake for 20 min until golden brown.
3. **Assembly:** Spread tomato sauce over crust, add bell pepper, red onion, mushrooms, cherry tomatoes, drizzle with olive oil.
4. **Topping Baking:** Bake for an additional 5 min until veggies are tender.
5. **Serving:** Garnish with fresh basil, slice, and serve.

Chef's Tips: *"Add garlic powder or red pepper flakes to crust for extra flavor. Use parchment paper to prevent sticking."*

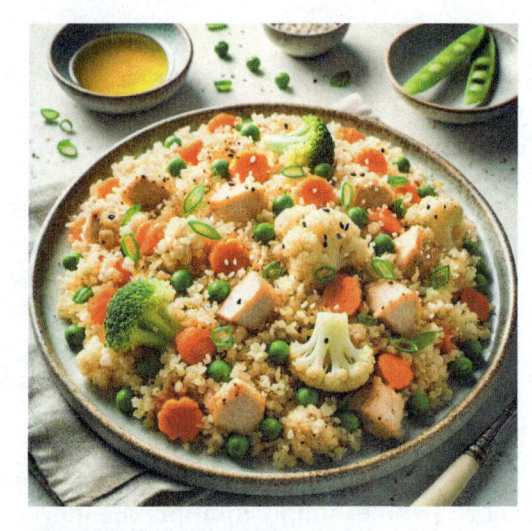

Nutritional Values: Calories: 300 kcal, Carbs: 18 g, Protein: 25 g, Fat: 15 g (Saturated Fat: 3 g, Monounsaturated Fat: 8 g, Polyunsaturated Fat: 2 g), Cholesterol: 140 mg, Sodium: 600 mg, Fiber: 5 g, Sugars: 4 g

Glycemic Index: Chicken breast: Low (GI = 0), Cauliflower: Very Low (GI = 15), Carrots: Low (GI = 35), Peas: Low (GI = 22), Eggs: Low (GI = 0)

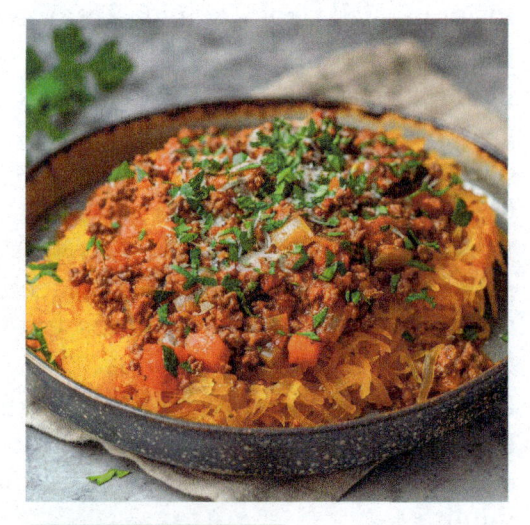

62. Spaghetti Squash Bolognese

Prep: 15 min | **Cook:** 45 min | **Total:** 60 min | **Difficulty:** 3/5

Ingredients: Spaghetti squash: 1 medium (800g, 28.22 oz), Ground beef: 300g (10.58 oz), Onion: 1 medium (150g, 5.29 oz), Carrots: 1 cup (130g, 4.59 oz), Celery: 1 cup (100g, 3.53 oz), Garlic: 2 cloves (6g, 0.21 oz), Crushed tomatoes: 2 cups (480g, 16.93 oz), Olive oil: 2 tbsp (30 ml, 1.01 oz), Oregano: 1 tsp (1g, 0.04 oz), Basil: 1 tsp (1g, 0.04 oz), Salt and pepper: to taste, Parsley: 2 tbsp (8g, 0.28 oz)

1. **Preparation:** Preheat the oven to 400°F (200°C). Halve squash, scoop seeds. Dice onion, carrots, celery. Mince garlic.
2. **Baking:** Place squash cut side down on a baking sheet. Bake for 35-40 min until tender. Scrape flesh into strands.
3. **Cooking:** Heat olive oil in a skillet. Sauté onion, carrots, celery, garlic 5 min. Add beef, brown.
4. **Sauce:** Stir in tomatoes, oregano, basil, salt, pepper. Simmer for 20 min.
5. **Serving:** Serve sauce over squash strands. Garnish with parsley.

Chef's Tips: *"For added flavor, sprinkle with grated Parmesan cheese or red pepper flakes."*

Nutritional Values: Calories: 350 kcal, Carbs: 25 g, Protein: 20 g, Fat: 18 g (Saturated Fat: 6 g, Monounsaturated Fat: 8 g, Polyunsaturated Fat: 2 g), Cholesterol: 60 mg, Sodium: 400 mg, Fiber: 6 g, Sugars: 13 g

Glycemic Index: Spaghetti squash: Low (GI = 41), Ground beef: Low (GI = 0), Crushed tomatoes: Low (GI = 15), Carrots: Low (GI = 35), Celery: Very Low (GI = 15)

63. Eggplant Lasagna with Ricotta and Mozzarella

Prep: 15 min | **Cook:** 40 min | **Total:** 55 min | **Difficulty:** 3/5

Ingredients: Eggplant: 2 large (600g, 21.16 oz), Ricotta: 1 cup (250g, 8.82 oz), Mozzarella: 1 cup (120g, 4.23 oz), Parmesan: 1/2 cup (50g, 1.76 oz), Marinara sauce: 2 cups (480g, 16.93 oz), Olive oil: 2 tbsp (30 ml, 1.01 oz), Basil: 2 tbsp (8g, 0.28 oz), Garlic: 2 cloves (6g, 0.21 oz), Salt and pepper: to taste

1.Preparation: Preheat the oven to 375°F (190°C). Slice eggplant, mince garlic.
2.Cooking: Brush eggplant with olive oil, season. Roast for 20 min, flip halfway.
3.Assembly: Layer marinara, eggplant, ricotta, garlic, mozzarella, Parmesan in a baking dish. Repeat, top with marinara, mozzarella, Parmesan.
4.Baking: Cover with foil, bake for 20 min. Remove foil, bake for 10 min.
5.Serving: Garnish with basil. Serve hot.

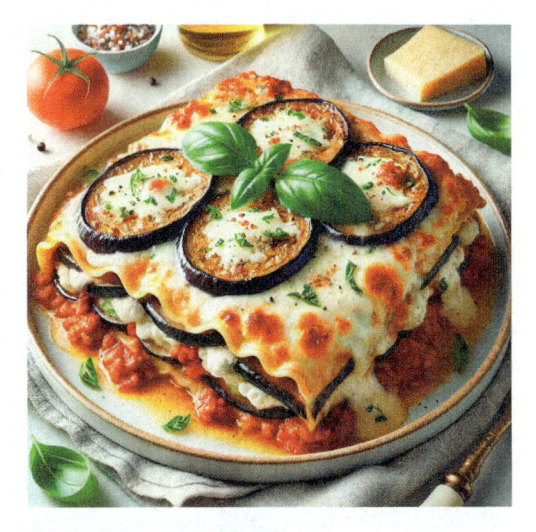

Nutritional Values: Calories: 400 kcal, Carbs: 20 g, Protein: 25 g, Fat: 25 g (Saturated Fat: 12 g, Monounsaturated Fat: 10 g, Polyunsaturated Fat: 3 g), Cholesterol: 70 mg, Sodium: 700 mg, Fiber: 8 g, Sugars: 8 g

Glycemic Index: Eggplant: Very Low (GI = 15), Ricotta: Low (GI = 30), Mozzarella: Low (GI = 30), Parmesan: Low (GI = 30), Marinara sauce: Low (GI = 30)

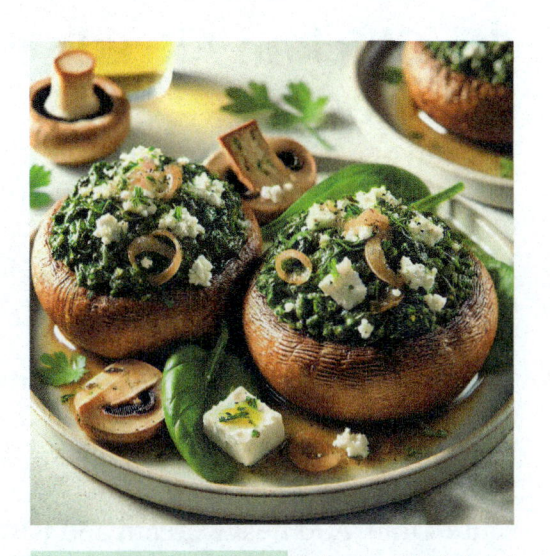

Chef's Tips: *"For added flavor, add a layer of sautéed spinach or mushrooms between the layers of eggplant."*

64. Stuffed Portobello Mushrooms with Spinach and Feta

Prep: 10 min | **Cook:** 20 min | **Total:** 30 min | **Difficulty:** 2/5

Ingredients: Portobello mushrooms: 4 large (400g, 14.11 oz), Fresh spinach, chopped: 2 cups (60g, 2.12 oz), Feta cheese, crumbled: 1/2 cup (75g, 2.65 oz), Olive oil: 2 tbsp (30 ml, 1.01 oz), Garlic, minced: 2 cloves (6g, 0.21 oz), Onion, diced: 1 small (100g, 3.53 oz), Salt and pepper: to taste, Fresh parsley, chopped: 2 tbsp (8g, 0.28 oz)

1.Preparation: Preheat the oven to 375°F (190°C). Remove stems from mushrooms and chop. Mince garlic and dice onion.
2.Cooking: Heat 1 tbsp olive oil in a skillet over medium heat. Sauté garlic and onion for 3-4 minutes until softened. Add chopped mushroom stems and spinach, cook until wilted. Season with salt and pepper.
3.Assembly: Place mushroom caps on a baking sheet. Fill each with spinach mixture and top with crumbled feta.
4.Baking: Drizzle with remaining olive oil. Bake for 15-20 minutes until mushrooms are tender and cheese is golden.
5.Serving: Garnish with chopped parsley. Serve hot.

Nutritional Values: Calories: 200 kcal, Carbs: 10 g, Protein: 10 g, Fat: 14 g (Saturated Fat: 4 g, Monounsaturated Fat: 8 g, Polyunsaturated Fat: 2 g), Cholesterol: 20 mg, Sodium: 400 mg, Fiber: 3 g, Sugars: 2 g

Glycemic Index: Portobello mushrooms: Very Low (GI = 15), Spinach: Very Low (GI = 15), Feta cheese: Low (GI = 30)

Chef's Tips: *"For added flavor, sprinkle with a pinch of red pepper flakes before baking."*

65. Cauliflower Crust Pizza with Veggie Toppings

Prep: 20 min | **Cook:** 25 min | **Total:** 45 min | **Difficulty:** 3/5

Ingredients: Cauliflower (riced): 1 medium head (600g), Mozzarella cheese: 1 cup (100g), Parmesan cheese: 1/4 cup (25g), Egg: 1, Italian seasoning: 1 tsp, Salt: 1/2 tsp, Black pepper: 1/2 tsp, Olive oil: 1 tbsp, Tomato sauce: 1/2 cup, Bell pepper (sliced): 1/2 cup, Red onion (sliced): 1/4 cup, Mushrooms (sliced): 1/2 cup, Cherry tomatoes (halved): 1/2 cup, Fresh basil: 2 tbsp

1. **Preparation:** Preheat oven to 400°F (200°C), line a baking sheet with parchment paper, steam riced cauliflower until tender, squeeze out moisture, mix cauliflower, mozzarella, Parmesan, egg, Italian seasoning, salt, and pepper.
2. **Crust Baking:** Form mixture into a crust on the baking sheet, bake for 20 min until golden brown.
3. **Assembly:** Spread tomato sauce over crust, add bell pepper, red onion, mushrooms, cherry tomatoes, drizzle with olive oil.
4. **Final Baking:** Bake for an additional 5 min until veggies are tender.
5. **Serving:** Garnish with fresh basil, slice, and serve.

Chef's Tips: *"Add garlic powder or red pepper flakes to crust for extra flavor. Use parchment paper to prevent sticking."*

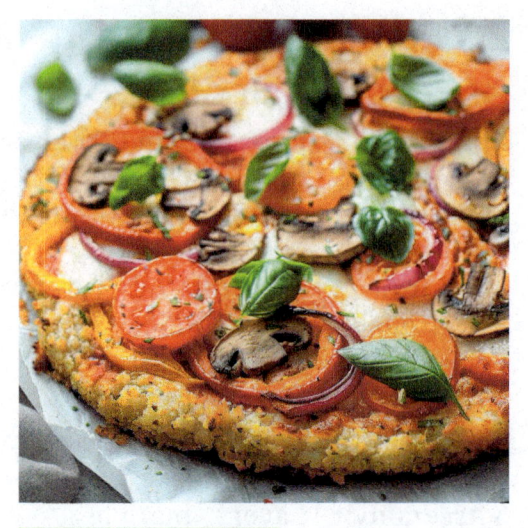

Nutritional Values: Calories: 300 kcal, Carbs: 18 g, Protein: 20 g, Fat: 18 g (Saturated Fat: 8 g, Monounsaturated Fat: 7 g, Polyunsaturated Fat: 3 g), Cholesterol: 70 mg, Sodium: 600 mg, Fiber: 6 g, Sugars: 8 g

Glycemic Index: Cauliflower: Very Low (GI = 15), Mozzarella: Low (GI = 30), Parmesan: Low (GI = 30), Bell peppers: Low (GI = 15), Cherry tomatoes: Low (GI = 15), Red onion: Low (GI = 10)

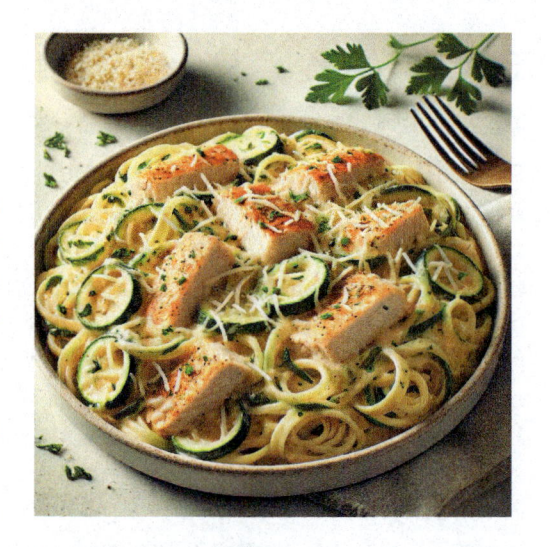

66. Chicken Alfredo with Zucchini Noodles

Prep: 10 min | **Cook:** 20 min | **Total:** 30 min | **Difficulty:** 2/5

Ingredients: Chicken breast: 300g (10.58 oz), Zucchini: 4 cups (600g, 21.16 oz), Olive oil: 2 tbsp (30 ml, 1.01 oz), Garlic: 2 cloves (6g, 0.21 oz), Heavy cream: 1 cup (240 ml), Parmesan: 1/2 cup (50g, 1.76 oz), Parsley: 2 tbsp (8g, 0.28 oz), Salt and pepper: to taste

1. **Preparation:** Dice chicken, spiralize zucchini, mince garlic.
2. **Cooking:** Heat 1 tbsp olive oil in a skillet. Cook chicken until browned, 5-7 min. Remove chicken.
3. **Sauce:** In the same skillet, add remaining olive oil and garlic, sauté 1 min. Add heavy cream and Parmesan, stir until smooth.
4. **Mixing:** Add zucchini noodles and chicken. Toss to coat with sauce, cook 2-3 min.
5. **Serving:** Season with salt and pepper. Garnish with parsley. Serve hot.

Chef's Tips: *"For extra flavor, add a pinch of red pepper flakes or a squeeze of lemon juice before serving."*

Nutritional Values: Calories: 350 kcal, Carbs: 12 g, Protein: 30 g, Fat: 22 g (Saturated Fat: 10 g, Monounsaturated Fat: 8 g, Polyunsaturated Fat: 2 g), Cholesterol: 100 mg, Sodium: 400 mg, Fiber: 4 g, Sugars: 4 g

Glycemic Index: Chicken breast: Low (GI = 0), Zucchini: Very Low (GI = 15), Heavy cream: Low (GI = 30), Parmesan cheese: Low (GI = 30)

SNACKS & SIDES

Healthy Snacks

Note: These recipes are designed for one serving. To accommodate more people, simply multiply the ingredients by the desired number of servings.

The words "tablespoon" and "teaspoon" have been shortened to "tbsp" and "tsp".

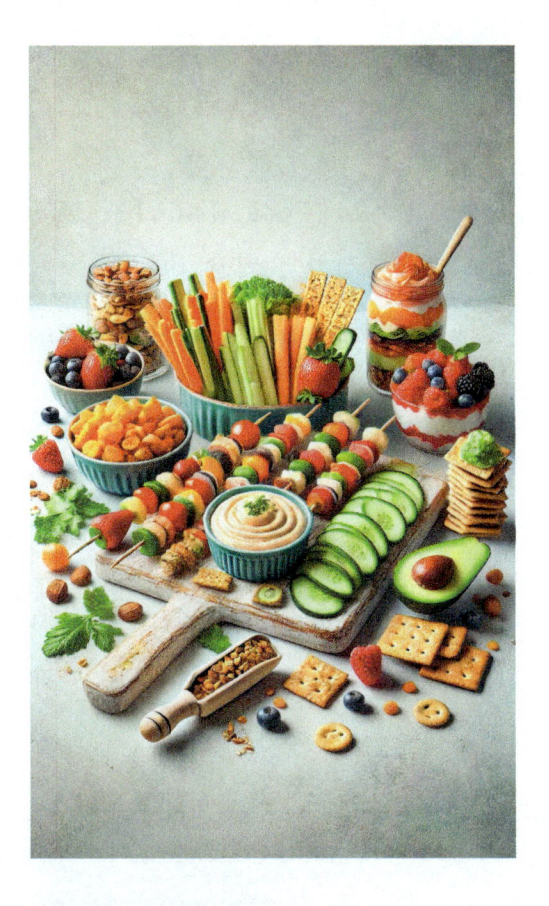

67. Cucumber Slices with Hummus

Prep: 10 min | **Cook:** 0 min | **Total:** 10 min | **Difficulty:** 1/5

Ingredients: Cucumber: 1 large (300g), Hummus: 1/2 cup (120g), Paprika: 1/2 tsp, Olive oil: 1 tsp (optional)

1. **Preparation:** Wash cucumber, slice into rounds.
2. **Assembly:** Arrange cucumber slices on a plate, top each with a small dollop of hummus, sprinkle with paprika.
3. **Serving:** Drizzle with olive oil if desired, serve immediately

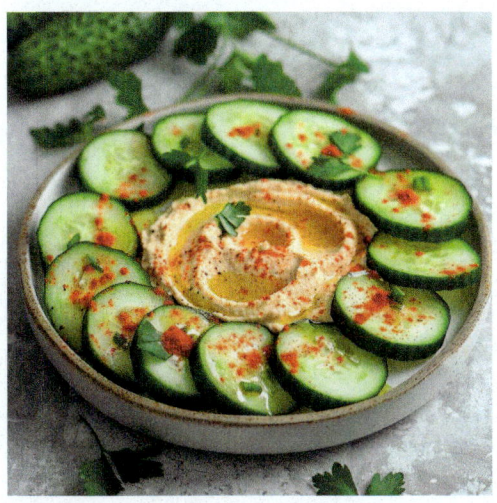

Nutritional Values: Calories: 120 kcal, Carbs: 15 g, Protein: 4 g, Fat: 6 g (Saturated Fat: 1 g, Monounsaturated Fat: 2 g, Polyunsaturated Fat: 3 g), Cholesterol: 0 mg, Sodium: 300 mg, Fiber: 4 g, Sugars: 3 g

Glycemic Index: Cucumber: Very Low (GI = 15), Hummus: Low (GI = 30)

Chef's Tips: *"For extra flavor, add a squeeze of lemon juice to the hummus. Use a variety of vegetables like bell pepper slices or carrot sticks as alternatives."*

68. Almond and Coconut Energy Balls

Prep: 10 min | **Cook:** 0 min | **Total:** 10 min | **Difficulty:** 1/5

Ingredients: Almonds, ground: 1 cup (120g, 4.23 oz), Shredded coconut: 1/2 cup (40g, 1.41 oz), Medjool dates, pitted: 10 (200g, 7.05 oz), Coconut oil: 2 tbsp (30 ml, 1.01 oz), Vanilla extract: 1 tsp (5 ml), Salt: a pinch

1. **Preparation:** In a food processor, blend almonds, shredded coconut, dates, coconut oil, vanilla extract, and salt until a sticky dough forms.
2. **Shaping:** Roll the mixture into small balls, about 1 inch in diameter.
3. **Serving:** Place the energy balls on a plate and refrigerate for 30 minutes before serving.

Chef's Tips: *"For added flavor, roll the energy balls in extra shredded coconut or cocoa powder before refrigerating."*

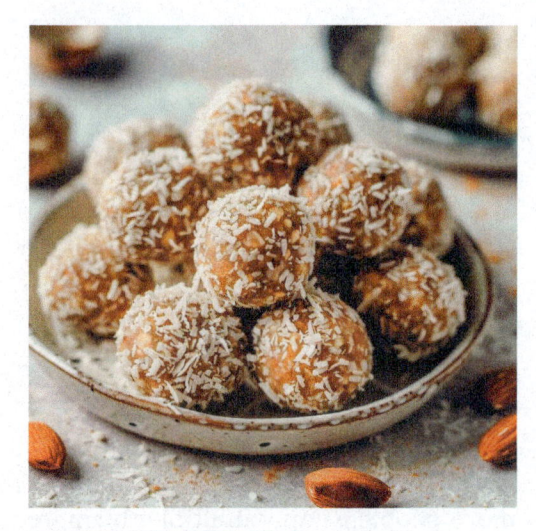

Nutritional Values: Calories: 120 kcal, Carbs: 14 g, Protein: 2 g, Fat: 7 g (Saturated Fat: 3 g, Monounsaturated Fat: 2 g, Polyunsaturated Fat: 1 g), Cholesterol: 0 mg, Sodium: 20 mg, Fiber: 3 g, Sugars: 13 g

Glycemic Index: Almonds: Very Low (GI = 15), Shredded coconut: Very Low (GI = 10), Dates: Medium (GI = 42)

69. Apple Slices with Almond Butter

Prep: 5 min | **Cook:** 0 min | **Total:** 5 min | **Difficulty:** 1/5

Ingredients: Apple: 1 large (200g, 7.05 oz), Almond butter: 2 tbsp (30g, 1.06 oz)

1. **Preparation:** Wash and core the apple, slice into thin wedges.
2. **Assembly:** Spread almond butter onto each apple slice.
3. **Serving:** Arrange on a plate, serve immediately.

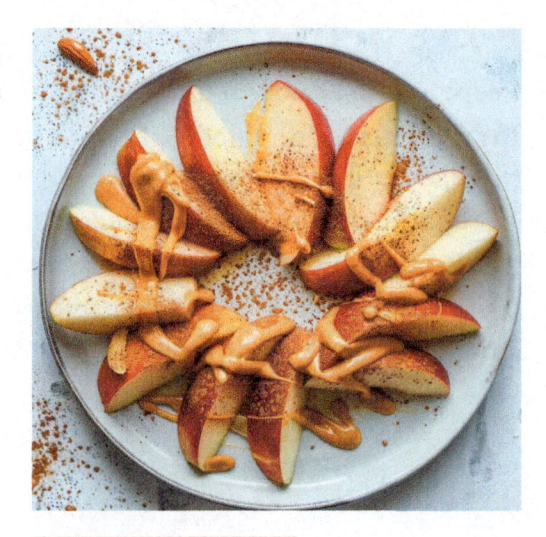

Chef's Tips: *"Add a sprinkle of cinnamon for extra flavor. Use natural almond butter with no added sugar for a healthier option."*

Nutritional Values: Calories: 150 kcal, Carbs: 20 g, Protein: 3 g, Fat: 7 g (Saturated Fat: 1 g, Monounsaturated Fat: 4 g, Polyunsaturated Fat: 2 g), Cholesterol: 0 mg, Sodium: 0 mg, Fiber: 4 g, Sugars: 19 g

Glycemic Index: Apple: Medium (GI = 39), Almond butter: Low (GI = 25)

70. Veggie Sticks with Guacamole

Prep: 10 min | **Cook:** 0 min | **Total:** 10 min | **Difficulty:** 1/5

Ingredients: Carrots, sliced into sticks: 1 cup (130g, 4.59 oz), Cucumbers, sliced into sticks: 1 cup (150g, 5.29 oz), Bell peppers, sliced into sticks: 1 cup (150g, 5.29 oz)

For the guacamole: Avocado: 2 medium (300g, 10.58 oz), Red onion, finely chopped: 1/4 cup (37.5g, 1.32 oz), Cilantro, chopped: 2 tbsp (8g, 0.28 oz), Lime juice: 2 tbsp (30 ml, 1.01 oz), Salt and pepper: to taste

1. Preparation: Slice carrots, cucumbers, and bell peppers into sticks. In a bowl, mash avocados with a fork. Stir in red onion, cilantro, lime juice, salt, and pepper.

2. Serving: Arrange veggie sticks on a plate and serve with a bowl of guacamole.

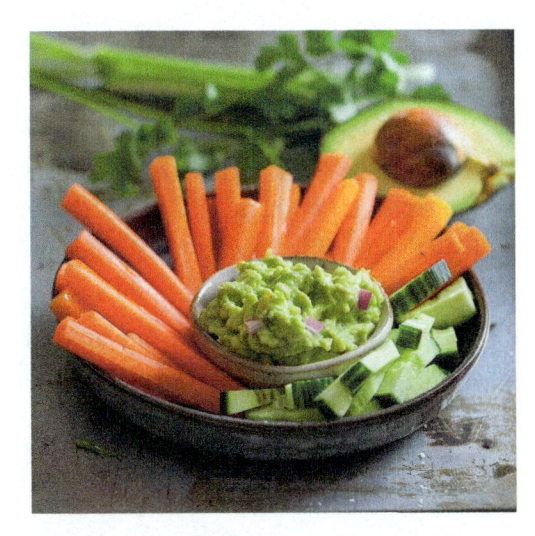

Nutritional Values: Calories: 200 kcal, Carbs: 18 g, Protein: 3 g, Fat: 15 g (Saturated Fat: 2 g, Monounsaturated Fat: 10 g, Polyunsaturated Fat: 2 g), Cholesterol: 0 mg, Sodium: 200 mg, Fiber: 8 g, Sugars: 4 g

Glycemic Index: Carrots: Low (GI = 35), Cucumbers: Very Low (GI = 15), Bell peppers: Low (GI = 15), Avocado: Very Low (GI = 15)

Chef's Tips: *"For extra flavor, add a pinch of garlic powder or chopped jalapeño to the guacamole."*

71. Whole Grain Crackers with Cream Cheese

Prep: 5 min | **Cook:** 0 min | **Total:** 5 min | **Difficulty:** 1/5

Ingredients: Whole grain crackers: 6 pieces (30g), Light cream cheese: 2 tbsp (30g)

1. Preparation: Spread light cream cheese evenly on each cracker.

2. Assembly: Arrange the crackers on a plate.

3. Serving: Serve immediately, garnish with a sprinkle of fresh herbs if desired.

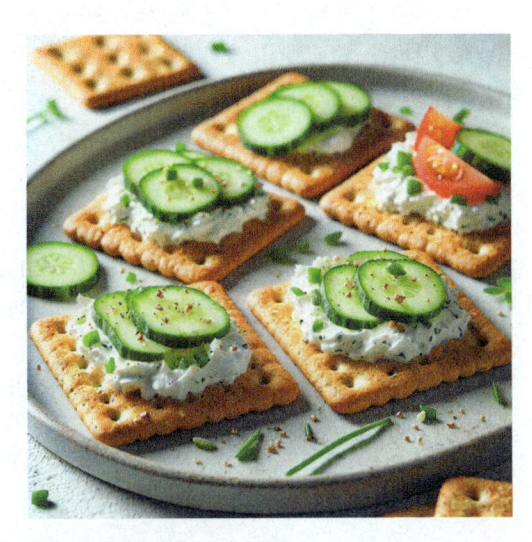

Nutritional Values: Calories: 200 kcal, Carbs: 20 g, Protein: 6 g, Fat: 10 g (Saturated Fat: 4 g, Monounsaturated Fat: 3 g, Polyunsaturated Fat: 2 g), Cholesterol: 20 mg, Sodium: 300 mg, Fiber: 4 g, Sugars: 1 g

Glycemic Index: Whole grain crackers: Medium (GI = 55), Light cream cheese: Low (GI = 30)

Chef's Tips: *"For added flavor, sprinkle with chopped fresh herbs like chives or parsley, or add a slice of cucumber or tomato on top."*

72. Berry and Nut Mix

Prep: 5 min | **Cook:** 0 min | **Total:** 5 min | **Difficulty:** 1/5

Ingredients: Mixed berries (strawberries, blueberries, raspberries): 1 cup (150g, 5.29 oz), Mixed nuts (almonds, walnuts, cashews): 1/2 cup (60g, 2.12 oz)

1. **Preparation:** Wash and dry the berries.
2. **Mixing:** Combine mixed berries and mixed nuts in a bowl.
3. **Serving:** Serve immediately or store in an airtight container for a quick snack.

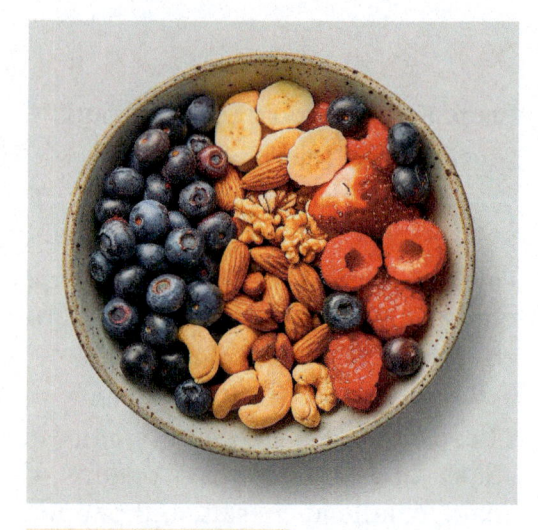

Nutritional Values: Calories: 200 kcal, Carbs: 20 g, Protein: 5 g, Fat: 12 g (Saturated Fat: 1.5 g, Monounsaturated Fat: 7 g, Polyunsaturated Fat: 3.5 g), Cholesterol: 0 mg, Sodium: 5 mg, Fiber: 6 g, Sugars: 12 g (from berries)

Chef's Tips: *"For added flavor, sprinkle a pinch of cinnamon or a drizzle of lemon juice over the mix."*

Glycemic Index: Mixed berries: Low (GI = 25), Mixed nuts: Very Low (GI = 15)

73. Baked Zucchini Chips

Prep: 10 min | **Cook:** 20 min | **Total:** 30 min | **Difficulty:** 2/5

Ingredients: Zucchini: 2 medium (400g), Olive oil: 1 tbsp (15ml), Salt: 1/2 tsp (2.5g), Pepper: 1/4 tsp (1.25g)

1. **Preparation:** Preheat oven to 225°C (450°F), slice zucchini thinly.
2. **Cooking:** Toss zucchini slices in olive oil, salt, and pepper, lay them in a single layer on a baking sheet, bake for 20 minutes or until crispy.
3. **Assembly:** Remove from oven and let cool slightly.
4. **Serving:** Serve warm or at room temperature as a healthy, crunchy snack.

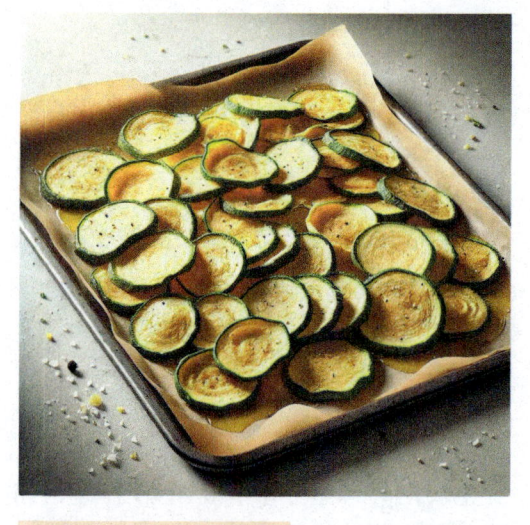

Nutritional Values: Calories: 80 kcal, Carbohydrates: 6g, Protein: 1g, Fat: 5g, Saturated Fat: 1g, Monounsaturated Fat: 3g, Polyunsaturated Fat: 1g, Cholesterol: 0mg, Sodium: 300mg, Fiber: 2g, Sugars: 3g (from zucchini)

Chef's Tips: *"Sprinkle with a little paprika or garlic powder for extra flavor."*

Glycemic Index: Zucchini: Very Low (GI = 15), Olive oil: Very Low (GI = 0)

SNACKS & SIDES

Sides to Share

Note: These recipes are designed for one serving. To accommodate more people, simply multiply the ingredients by the desired number of servings.

The words "tablespoon" and "teaspoon" have been shortened to "tbsp" and "tsp".

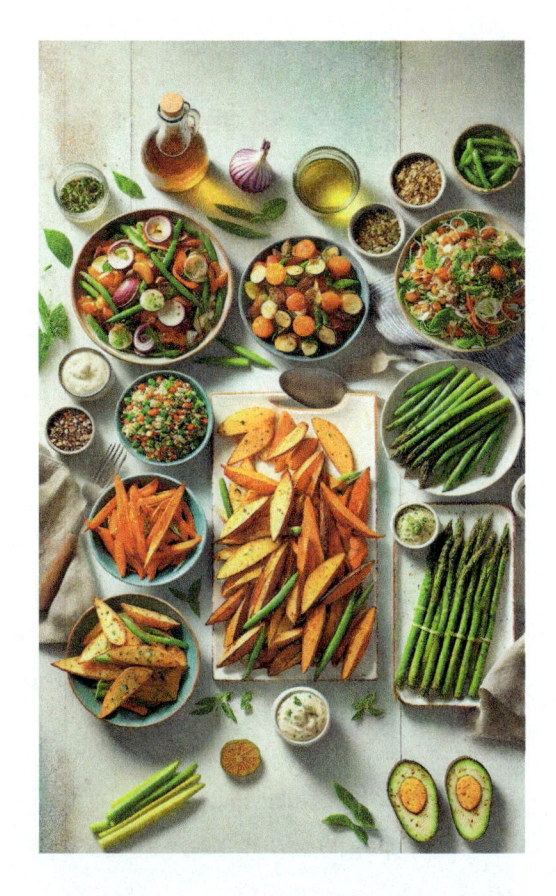

74. Garlic and Herb Roasted Brussels Sprout

Prep: 10 min | **Cook:** 25 min | **Total:** 35 min | **Difficulty:** 2/5

Ingredients: Brussels sprouts, halved: 4 cups (600g, 21.16 oz), Olive oil: 2 tbsp (30 ml, 1.01 oz), Garlic, minced: 2 cloves (6g, 0.21 oz), Fresh rosemary, chopped: 1 tbsp (4g, 0.14 oz), Fresh thyme, chopped: 1 tbsp (4g, 0.14 oz), Salt and pepper: to taste

1.Preparation: Preheat the oven to 400°F (200°C). Halve the Brussels sprouts and mince the garlic.

2.Mixing: In a large bowl, toss the Brussels sprouts with olive oil, garlic, rosemary, thyme, salt, and pepper.

3.Cooking: Spread the Brussels sprouts on a baking sheet in a single layer. Roast in the preheated oven for 20-25 minutes until tender and golden brown, stirring halfway through.

4.Serving: Serve hot, garnished with additional fresh herbs if desired.

Chef's Tips: *"For added flavor, sprinkle with grated Parmesan cheese or a drizzle of balsamic glaze before serving."*

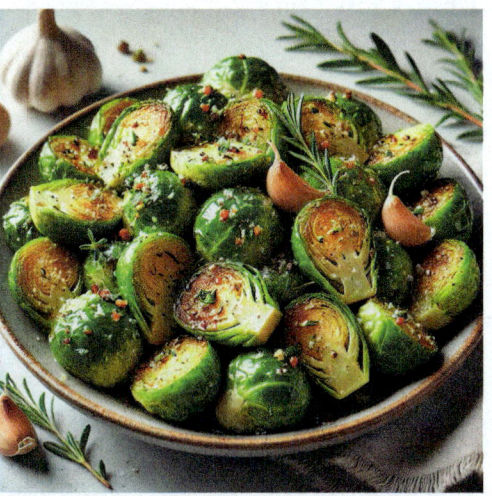

Nutritional Values: Calories: 180 kcal, Carbs: 18 g, Protein: 5 g, Fat: 10 g (Saturated Fat: 1.5 g, Monounsaturated Fat: 6 g, Polyunsaturated Fat: 1.5 g), Cholesterol: 0 mg, Sodium: 200 mg, Fiber: 7 g, Sugars: 4 g (from Brussels sprouts)

Glycemic Index: Brussels sprouts: Very Low (GI = 15)

75. Quinoa Pilaf with Fresh Herbs

Prep: 10 min | **Cook:** 20 min | **Total:** 30 min | **Difficulty:** 2/5

Ingredients: Quinoa: 1 cup (170g, 6 oz), Vegetable broth: 2 cups (480 ml), Olive oil: 1 tbsp (15 ml, 0.51 oz), Onion, finely chopped: 1 small (100g, 3.53 oz), Garlic, minced: 2 cloves (6g, 0.21 oz), Fresh parsley, chopped: 2 tbsp (8g, 0.28 oz), Fresh cilantro, chopped: 2 tbsp (8g, 0.28 oz), Fresh mint, chopped: 1 tbsp (4g, 0.14 oz), Lemon juice: 1 tbsp (15 ml, 0.51 oz), Salt and pepper: to taste

1.Preparation: Rinse quinoa under cold water. Finely chop onion and garlic.

2.Cooking: Heat olive oil in a saucepan over medium heat. Sauté onion and garlic for 3-4 minutes until softened. Add quinoa and cook for 2 minutes, stirring constantly.

3.Simmering: Add vegetable broth, bring to a boil. Reduce heat to low, cover, and simmer for 15 minutes until quinoa is tender and liquid is absorbed.

4.Mixing: Remove from heat, fluff with a fork. Stir in parsley, cilantro, mint, lemon juice, salt, and pepper.

5.Serving: Serve hot as a side dish.

Chef's Tips: *"For added flavor, toast the quinoa in the saucepan for a few minutes before adding the vegetable broth."*

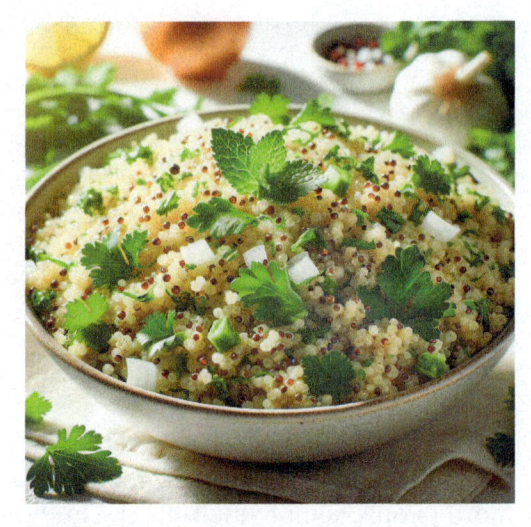

Nutritional Values: Calories: 200 kcal, Carbs: 30 g, Protein: 5 g, Fat: 6 g (Saturated Fat: 0.5 g, Monounsaturated Fat: 4 g, Polyunsaturated Fat: 1.5 g), Cholesterol: 0 mg, Sodium: 300 mg, Fiber: 4 g, Sugars: 1 g

Glycemic Index: Quinoa: Low (GI = 53)

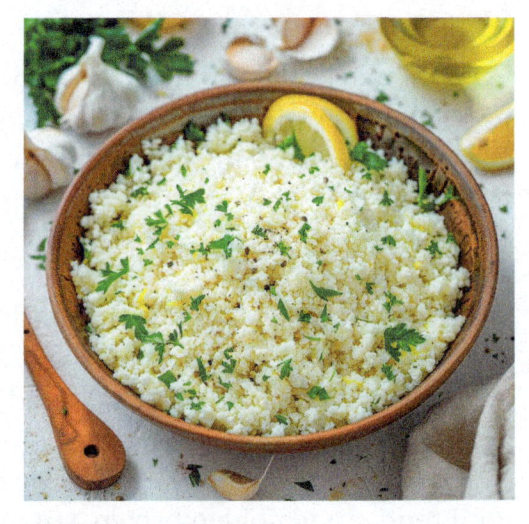

76. Cauliflower Rice with Lemon and Parsley

Prep: 10 min | **Cook:** 10 min | **Total:** 20 min | **Difficulty:** 1/5

Ingredients: Cauliflower, riced: 4 cups (600g, 21.16 oz), Olive oil: 2 tbsp (30 ml, 1.01 oz), Garlic, minced: 2 cloves (6g, 0.21 oz), Lemon zest: 1 tsp (2g, 0.07 oz), Lemon juice: 2 tbsp (30 ml, 1.01 oz), Fresh parsley, chopped: 2 tbsp (8g, 0.28 oz), Salt and pepper: to taste

1.Preparation: Rice the cauliflower. Mince garlic and chop parsley.

2.Cooking: Heat olive oil in a large skillet over medium heat. Sauté garlic for 1 minute until fragrant. Add riced cauliflower and cook for 5-7 minutes until tender.

3.Mixing: Stir in lemon zest, lemon juice, salt, and pepper. Cook for an additional 2 minutes.

4.Serving: Remove from heat, stir in fresh parsley, and serve hot.

Chef's Tips: *"For added flavor, sprinkle with toasted pine nuts or grated Parmesan cheese before serving."*

Nutritional Values: Calories: 120 kcal, Carbs: 10 g, Protein: 3 g, Fat: 8 g (Saturated Fat: 1 g, Monounsaturated Fat: 5 g, Polyunsaturated Fat: 2 g), Cholesterol: 0 mg, Sodium: 150 mg, Fiber: 4 g, Sugars: 2 g

Glycemic Index: Cauliflower: Very Low (GI = 15)

77. Balsamic Glazed Carrots

Prep: 10 min | **Cook:** 20 min | **Total:** 30 min | **Difficulty:** 2/5

Ingredients: Carrots, peeled and sliced: 4 cups (600g, 21.16 oz), Olive oil: 2 tbsp (30 ml, 1.01 oz), Balsamic vinegar: 1/4 cup (60 ml, 2.12 oz), Honey substitute: 1 tbsp (15 ml, 0.51 oz), Garlic, minced: 2 cloves (6g, 0.21 oz), Fresh thyme, chopped: 1 tbsp (4g, 0.14 oz), Salt and pepper: to taste

1. **Preparation:** Peel and slice carrots. Mince garlic and chop thyme.
2. **Cooking:** Heat olive oil in a large skillet over medium heat. Add carrots and cook for 10-12 minutes until tender.
3. **Glazing:** Add balsamic vinegar, honey substitute, garlic, thyme, salt, and pepper. Cook for an additional 5-7 minutes, stirring frequently, until the carrots are glazed and the sauce has thickened.
4. **Serving:** Serve hot, garnished with additional fresh thyme if desired.

Chef's Tips: *"For added flavor, sprinkle with a pinch of red pepper flakes or a drizzle of lemon juice before serving."*

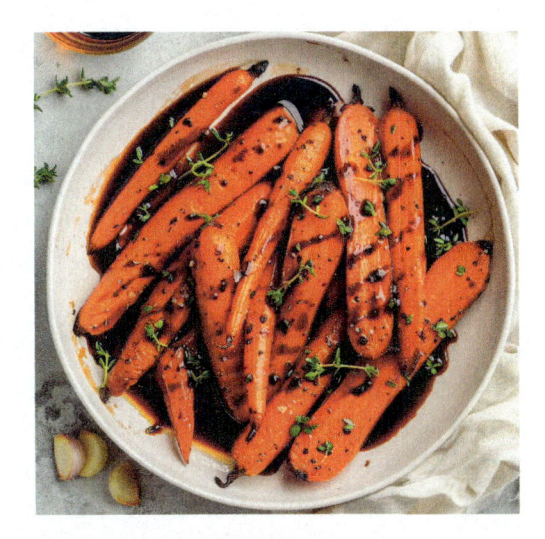

Nutritional Values: Calories: 140 kcal, Carbs: 22 g, Protein: 2 g, Fat: 6 g (Saturated Fat: 1 g, Monounsaturated Fat: 4 g, Polyunsaturated Fat: 1 g), Cholesterol: 0 mg, Sodium: 150 mg, Fiber: 6 g, Sugars: 8 g

Glycemic Index: Carrots: Low (GI = 35)

78. Green Bean Almondine

Prep: 10 min | **Cook:** 10 min | **Total:** 20 min | **Difficulty:** 2/5

Ingredients: Green beans, trimmed: 4 cups (600g, 21.16 oz), Sliced almonds: 1/2 cup (50g, 1.76 oz), Butter: 2 tbsp (30g, 1.06 oz), Garlic, minced: 2 cloves (6g, 0.21 oz), Lemon juice: 1 tbsp (15 ml, 0.51 oz), Fresh parsley, chopped: 2 tbsp (8g, 0.28 oz), Salt and pepper: to taste

1. **Preparation:** Trim green beans. Mince garlic and chop parsley.
2. **Cooking:** Bring a pot of salted water to a boil. Add green beans and cook for 3-4 minutes until tender-crisp. Drain and set aside.
3. **Sautéing:** In a large skillet, melt butter over medium heat. Add garlic and sliced almonds, sauté for 2-3 minutes until fragrant and almonds are golden brown. Add green beans, lemon juice, salt, and pepper. Toss to coat and cook for an additional 2 minutes.
4. **Serving:** Remove from heat, stir in fresh parsley, and serve hot.

Chef's Tips: *"For added flavor, sprinkle with grated Parmesan cheese or a pinch of red pepper flakes before serving."*

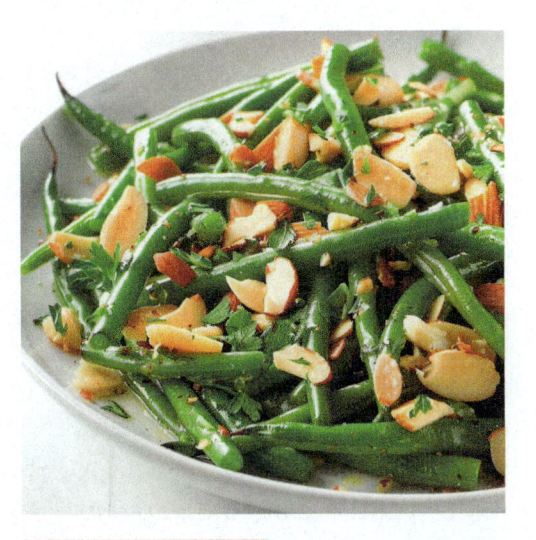

Nutritional Values: Calories: 180 kcal, Carbs: 12 g, Protein: 4 g, Fat: 14 g (Saturated Fat: 3 g, Monounsaturated Fat: 7 g, Polyunsaturated Fat: 3 g), Cholesterol: 10 mg, Sodium: 150 mg, Fiber: 6 g, Sugars: 2 g (from green beans)

Glycemic Index: Green beans: Very Low (GI = 15)

79. Roasted Sweet Potato Wedges

Prep: 10 min | **Cook:** 30 min | **Total:** 40 min | **Difficulty:** 1/5

Ingredients: Sweet potatoes, cut into wedges: 4 cups (600g, 21.16 oz), Olive oil: 2 tbsp (30 ml, 1.01 oz), Paprika: 1 tsp (2g, 0.07 oz), Garlic powder: 1 tsp (2g, 0.07 oz), Fresh rosemary, chopped: 1 tbsp (4g, 0.14 oz), Salt and pepper: to taste

1. **Preparation:** Preheat the oven to 400°F (200°C). Cut sweet potatoes into wedges. Chop rosemary.
2. **Mixing:** In a large bowl, toss sweet potato wedges with olive oil, paprika, garlic powder, rosemary, salt, and pepper.
3. **Cooking:** Spread the sweet potato wedges on a baking sheet in a single layer. Roast in the preheated oven for 25-30 minutes, flipping halfway through, until golden brown and tender.
4. **Serving:** Serve hot, garnished with additional fresh rosemary if desired.

Chef's Tips: *"For added flavor, drizzle with balsamic glaze or sprinkle with grated Parmesan cheese before serving."*

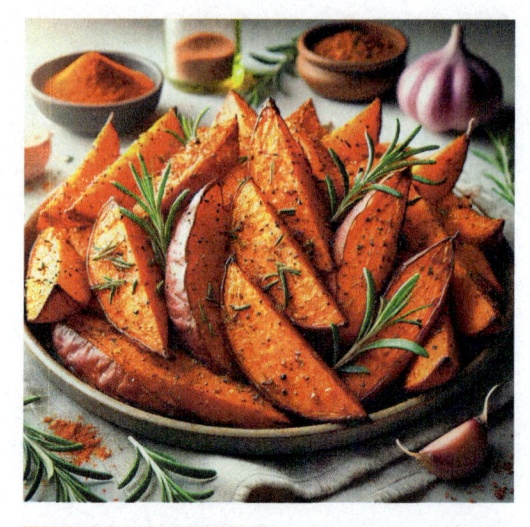

Nutritional Values: Calories: 180 kcal, Carbs: 30 g, Protein: 2 g, Fat: 7 g (Saturated Fat: 1 g, Monounsaturated Fat: 5 g, Polyunsaturated Fat: 1 g), Cholesterol: 0 mg, Sodium: 200 mg, Fiber: 4 g, Sugars: 8 g

Glycemic Index: Sweet potatoes: Medium (GI = 63)

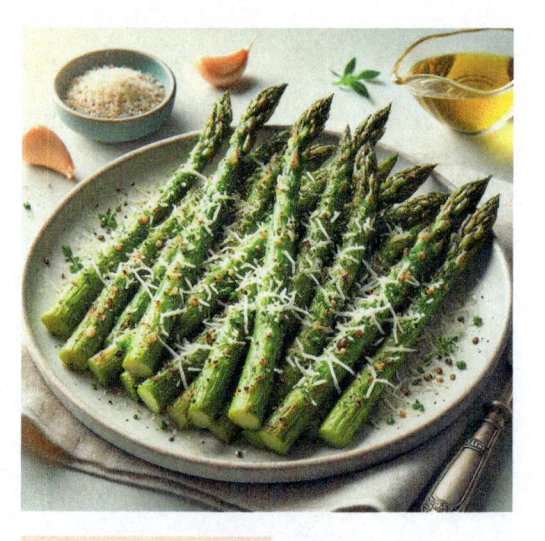

80. Garlic Parmesan Roasted Asparagus

Prep: 10 min | **Cook:** 15 min | **Total:** 25 min | **Difficulty:** 1/5

Ingredients: Asparagus, trimmed: 4 cups (600g, 21.16 oz), Olive oil: 2 tbsp (30 ml, 1.01 oz), Garlic, minced: 2 cloves (6g, 0.21 oz), Parmesan cheese, grated: 1/4 cup (25g, 0.88 oz), Salt and pepper: to taste

1. **Preparation:** Preheat the oven to 400°F (200°C). Trim the asparagus and mince the garlic.
2. **Mixing:** In a large bowl, toss the asparagus with olive oil, minced garlic, salt, and pepper.
3. **Cooking:** Spread the asparagus on a baking sheet in a single layer. Roast in the preheated oven for 12-15 minutes until tender and slightly crispy.
4. **Serving:** Remove from oven, sprinkle with grated Parmesan cheese. Serve hot.

Chef's Tips: *"For added flavor, drizzle with a squeeze of lemon juice or sprinkle with red pepper flakes before serving."*

Nutritional Values: Calories: 120 kcal, Carbs: 6 g, Protein: 5 g, Fat: 9 g (Saturated Fat: 2 g, Monounsaturated Fat: 5 g, Polyunsaturated Fat: 1 g), Cholesterol: 5 mg, Sodium: 200 mg, Fiber: 3 g, Sugars: 3 g (from asparagus)

Glycemic Index: Asparagus: Very Low (GI = 15)

DESSERTS & SWEET TREATS

Fruit-Based Desserts

Note: These recipes are designed for one serving. To accommodate more people, simply multiply the ingredients by the desired number of servings.

The words "tablespoon" and "teaspoon" have been shortened to "tbsp" and "tsp".

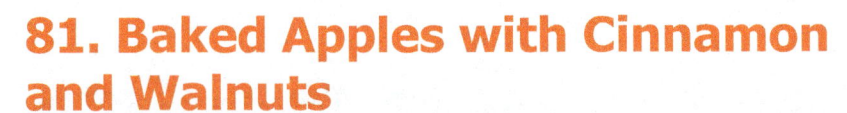

81. Baked Apples with Cinnamon and Walnuts

Prep: 10 min | **Cook:** 30 min | **Total:** 40 min | **Difficulty:** 2/5

Ingredients: Apples: 4 medium (600g, 21.16 oz), Walnuts, chopped: 1/2 cup (60g, 2.12 oz), Ground cinnamon: 2 tsp (4g, 0.14 oz), Unsweetened apple juice: 1/2 cup (120 ml), Lemon juice: 1 tbsp (15 ml, 0.51 oz), Butter, melted: 2 tbsp (30g, 1.06 oz)

1. Preparation: Preheat the oven to 375°F (190°C). Core the apples, leaving the bottoms intact.

2. Stuffing: In a bowl, mix chopped walnuts, ground cinnamon, and a little melted butter. Stuff the apples with this mixture.

3. Baking: Place the stuffed apples in a baking dish. Pour apple juice and lemon juice over them. Drizzle with remaining melted butter. Bake in the preheated oven for 30 minutes until the apples are tender.

4. Serving: Serve warm, optionally with a dollop of Greek yogurt or a sprinkle of extra cinnamon.

Chef's Tips: *"For added flavor, sprinkle with a pinch of nutmeg or add a few raisins to the walnut mixture."*

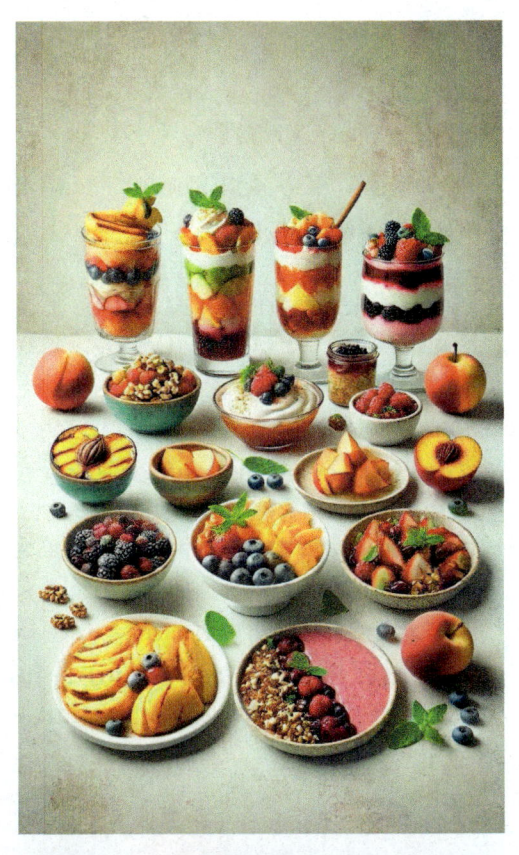

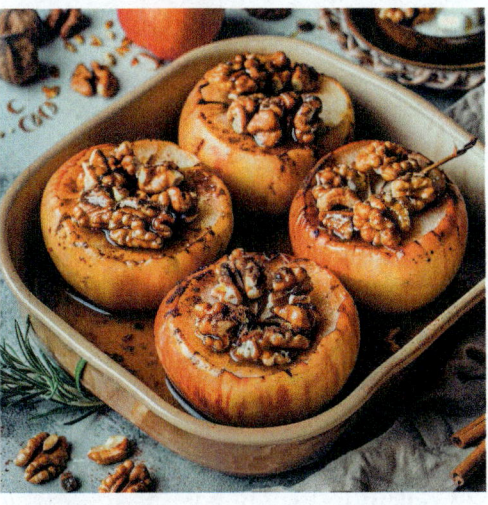

Nutritional Values: Calories: 200 kcal, Carbs: 30 g, Protein: 2 g, Fat: 10 g (Saturated Fat: 2 g, Monounsaturated Fat: 3 g, Polyunsaturated Fat: 4 g), Cholesterol: 10 mg, Sodium: 20 mg, Fiber: 6 g, Sugars: 30g (from apples)

Glycemic Index: Apples: Medium (GI = 39), Walnuts: Very Low (GI = 15)

82. Mixed Berry Compote with Greek Yogurt

Prep: 5 min | **Cook:** 10 min | **Total:** 15 min | **Difficulty:** 1/5

Ingredients: Mixed berries (strawberries, blueberries, raspberries): 2 cups (300g, 10.58 oz), Water: 1/4 cup (60 ml), Lemon juice: 1 tbsp (15 ml, 0.51 oz), Stevia: 1 tsp (4g, 0.14 oz), Greek yogurt: 1 cup (240g, 8.47 oz), Fresh mint, chopped: 1 tbsp (4g, 0.14 oz)

1. **Preparation:** Wash and drain the berries.
2. **Cooking:** In a small saucepan, combine berries, water, lemon juice, and stevia. Cook over medium heat for 10 minutes, stirring occasionally, until berries break down and the mixture thickens.
3. **Mixing:** Remove from heat and let cool slightly.
4. **Serving:** Spoon Greek yogurt into bowls and top with berry compote. Garnish with fresh mint.

Chef's Tips: *"For added texture, sprinkle with a handful of granola or chopped nuts before serving."*

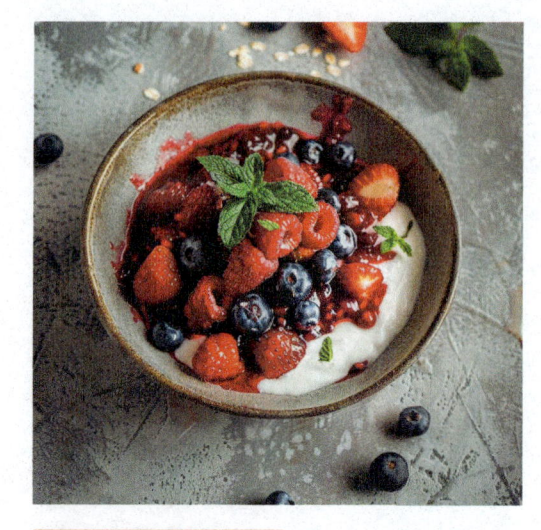

Nutritional Values: Calories: 150 kcal, Carbs: 20 g, Protein: 10 g, Fat: 4 g (Saturated Fat: 2 g, Monounsaturated Fat: 1 g, Polyunsaturated Fat: 0.5 g), Cholesterol: 10 mg, Sodium: 40 mg, Fiber: 4 g, Sugars: 15g (from mixed berries and Greek yogurt)

Glycemic Index: Mixed berries: Low (GI = 25), Greek yogurt: Low (GI = 30)

83. Grilled Peaches with Stevia and Mint

Prep: 5 min | **Cook:** 10 min | **Total:** 15 min | **Difficulty:** 1/5

Ingredients: Peaches, halved and pitted: 4 (600g, 21.16 oz), Stevia: 1 tsp (4g, 0.14 oz), Olive oil: 1 tbsp (15 ml, 0.51 oz), Fresh mint, chopped: 2 tbsp (8g, 0.28 oz)

1. **Preparation:** Preheat grill to medium-high heat. Halve and pit the peaches.
2. **Cooking:** Brush the peach halves with olive oil. Place the peaches cut side down on the grill. Cook for 4-5 minutes until grill marks appear. Flip the peaches and cook for an additional 3-4 minutes until tender.
3. **Assembly:** Remove peaches from the grill. Sprinkle with stevia.
4. **Serving:** Garnish with chopped fresh mint. Serve warm.

Chef's Tips: *"For added flavor, sprinkle with a pinch of cinnamon or a dollop of Greek yogurt before serving."*

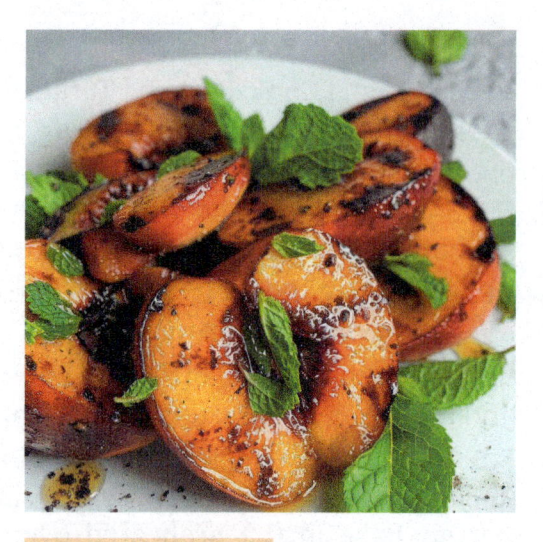

Nutritional Values: Calories: 100 kcal, Carbs: 20 g, Protein: 1 g, Fat: 2 g (Saturated Fat: 0 g, Monounsaturated Fat: 1 g, Polyunsaturated Fat: 0.5 g), Cholesterol: 0 mg, Sodium: 0 mg, Fiber: 3 g, Sugars: 15 g (from peaches)

Glycemic Index: Peaches: Medium (GI = 42), Stevia: Very Low (GI = 0)

84. Mango and Berry Parfait

Prep: 10 min | **Cook:** 0 min | **Total:** 10 min | **Difficulty:** 1/5

Ingredients: Mango, diced: 1 cup (150g, 5.29 oz), Mixed berries (strawberries, blueberries, raspberries): 1 cup (150g, 5.29 oz), Greek yogurt: 1 cup (240g, 8.47 oz), Stevia: 1 tsp (4g, 0.14 oz), Fresh mint, chopped: 1 tbsp (4g, 0.14 oz)

1. **Preparation:** Dice the mango and wash the berries.
2. **Assembly:** In a glass or bowl, layer Greek yogurt, diced mango, and mixed berries. Sprinkle stevia between layers.
3. **Serving:** Garnish with chopped fresh mint. Serve immediately.

Chef's Tips: *"For added texture, sprinkle with a handful of granola or chopped nuts before serving."*

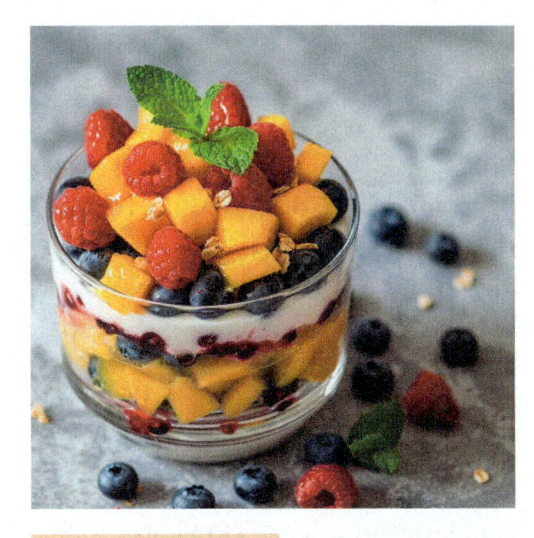

Nutritional Values: Calories: 180 kcal, Carbs: 30 g, Protein: 10 g, Fat: 2 g (Saturated Fat: 1 g, Monounsaturated Fat: 0.5 g, Polyunsaturated Fat: 0.5 g), Cholesterol: 5 mg, Sodium: 40 mg, Fiber: 4 g, Sugars: 30g (from mango and mixed berries)

Glycemic Index: Mango: Medium (GI = 51), Mixed berries: Low (GI = 25), Greek yogurt: Low (GI = 30), Stevia: Very Low (GI = 0)

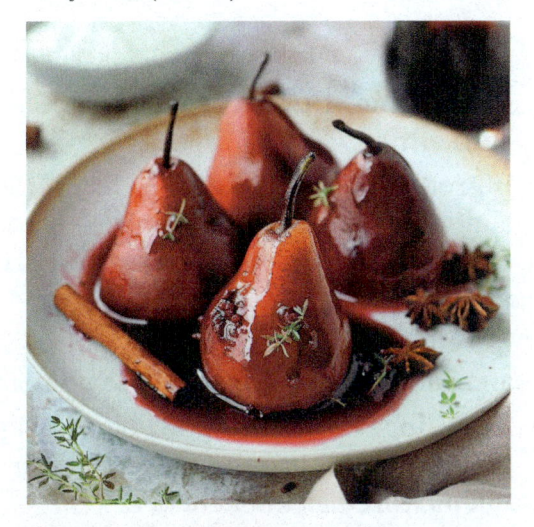

85. Poached Pears in Red Wine

Prep: 10 min | **Cook:** 30 min | **Total:** 40 min | **Difficulty:** 2/5

Ingredients: Pears, peeled and cored: 4 (800g, 28.22 oz), Dry red wine: 2 cups (480 ml), Water: 1 cup (240 ml), Stevia: 2 tsp (8g, 0.28 oz), Cinnamon stick: 1, Whole cloves: 4, Orange zest: 1 tbsp (6g, 0.21 oz)

1. **Preparation:** Peel and core the pears, keeping them whole.
2. **Cooking:** In a large saucepan, combine red wine, water, stevia, cinnamon stick, cloves, and orange zest. Bring to a simmer over medium heat.
3. **Poaching:** Add the pears to the saucepan. Simmer gently for 25-30 minutes, turning occasionally, until the pears are tender.
4. **Serving:** Remove pears from the liquid and let them cool slightly. Serve warm or chilled, with a drizzle of the poaching liquid.

Chef's Tips: *"For added flavor, serve with a dollop of Greek yogurt or a sprinkle of chopped nuts."*

Nutritional Values: Calories: 150 kcal, Carbs: 25 g, Protein: 1 g, Fat: 0 g (Saturated Fat: 0 g, Monounsaturated Fat: 0 g, Polyunsaturated Fat: 0 g), Cholesterol: 0 mg, Sodium: 5 mg, Fiber: 6 g, Sugars: 35 g (from pears and red wine)

Glycemic Index: Pears: Medium (GI = 38), Red wine: Low (GI = 0), Stevia: Very Low (GI = 0)

86. Tropical Fruit Salad with Lime and Coconut

Prep: 15 min | **Cook:** 0 min | **Total:** 15 min | **Difficulty:** 1/5

Ingredients: Mango, diced: 1 cup (150g, 5.29 oz), Pineapple, diced: 1 cup (150g, 5.29 oz), Kiwi, sliced: 2 (150g, 5.29 oz), Papaya, diced: 1 cup (150g, 5.29 oz), Shredded coconut: 1/4 cup (20g, 0.71 oz), Lime juice: 2 tbsp (30 ml, 1.01 oz), Fresh mint, chopped: 1 tbsp (4g, 0.14 oz)

1. **Preparation:** Dice the mango, pineapple, and papaya. Slice the kiwi.
2. **Mixing:** In a large bowl, combine the mango, pineapple, kiwi, and papaya. Drizzle with lime juice and toss gently.
3. **Serving:** Sprinkle with shredded coconut and chopped fresh mint. Serve immediately.

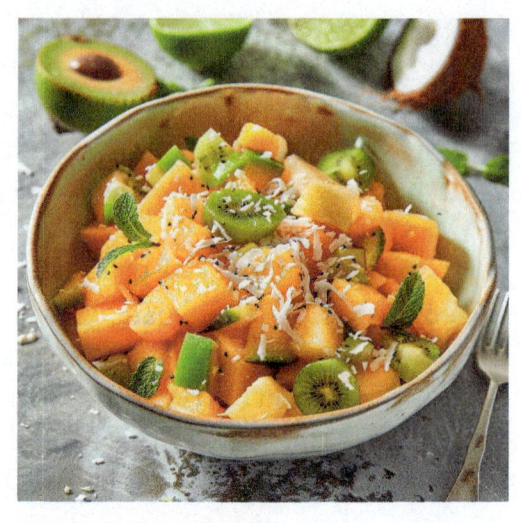

Nutritional Values: Calories: 150 kcal, Carbs: 35 g, Protein: 2 g, Fat: 2 g (Saturated Fat: 1.5 g, Monounsaturated Fat: 0.2 g, Polyunsaturated Fat: 0.1 g), Cholesterol: 0 mg, Sodium: 10 mg, Fiber: 5 g, Sugars: 30 g (from fruits)

Glycemic Index: Mango: Medium (GI = =51), Pineapple: Medium (GI = 66), Kiwi: Low (GI = 50), Papaya: Low (GI = 60), Shredded coconut: Very Low (GI = 10)

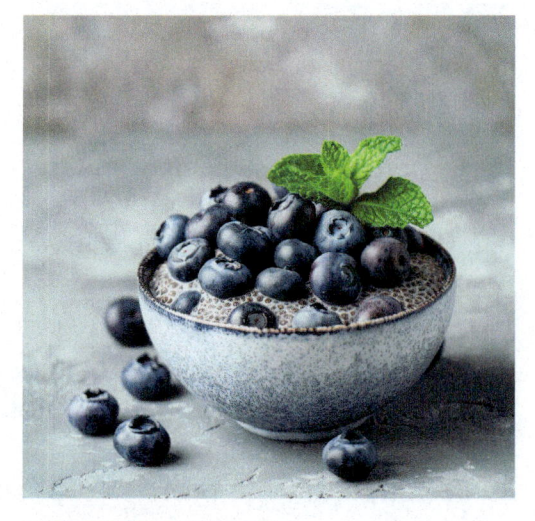

Chef's Tips: *"For added flavor, sprinkle a pinch of lime zest or a dash of chili powder over the fruit salad."*

87. Blueberry Chia Pudding

Prep: 5 min | **Cook:** 0 min | **Chill:** 4 hrs | **Total:** 4 hrs 5 min | **Difficulty:** 1/5

Ingredients: Chia seeds: 1/4 cup (50g, 1.76 oz), Unsweetened almond milk: 1 cup (240 ml), Stevia: 1 tsp (4g, 0.14 oz), Vanilla extract: 1 tsp (5 ml), Blueberries: 1 cup (150g, 5.29 oz), Fresh mint, chopped: 1 tbsp (4g, 0.14 oz)

1. **Preparation:** In a bowl, mix chia seeds, almond milk, stevia, and vanilla extract. Stir well to combine.
2. **Chilling:** Cover the bowl and refrigerate for at least 4 hours, or overnight, until the chia seeds have absorbed the liquid and the mixture has thickened.
3. **Serving:** Stir the chia pudding before serving. Top with blueberries and garnish with chopped fresh mint.

Nutritional Values: Calories: 150 kcal, Carbs: 20 g, Protein: 4 g, Fat: 7 g (Saturated Fat: 0.5 g, Monounsaturated Fat: 2 g, Polyunsaturated Fat: 4 g), Cholesterol: 0 mg, Sodium: 30 mg, Fiber: 8 g, Sugars: 12 g

Glycemic Index: Chia seeds: Very Low (GI = 1), Unsweetened almond milk: Very Low (GI = 30), Blueberries: Low (GI = 53)

Chef's Tips: *"For added texture and flavor, sprinkle with a handful of granola or nuts before serving."*

DESSERTS & SWEET TREATS

Diabetes-Friendly Baking

Note: These recipes are designed for one serving. To accommodate more people, simply multiply the ingredients by the desired number of servings.

The words "tablespoon" and "teaspoon" have been shortened to "tbsp" and "tsp".

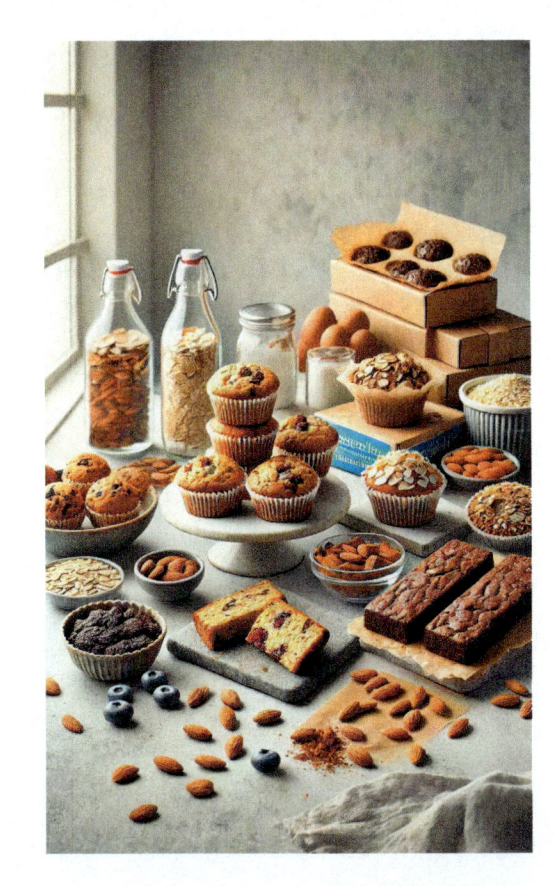

88. Almond Flour Blueberry Muffins

Prep: 10 min | **Cook:** 20 min | **Total:** 30 min | **Difficulty:** 2/5

Ingredients: Almond flour: 2 cups (200g, 7.05 oz), Eggs: 3 large, Blueberries: 1 cup (150g, 5.29 oz), Stevia: 2 tbsp (8g, 0.28 oz), Baking powder: 1 tsp (4g, 0.14 oz), Vanilla extract: 1 tsp (5 ml), Unsweetened almond milk: 1/2 cup (120 ml), Coconut oil, melted: 1/4 cup (60 ml, 2.12 oz), Salt: a pinch

1. Preparation: Preheat the oven to 350°F (175°C). Line a muffin tin with paper liners.

2. Mixing: In a large bowl, whisk together almond flour, stevia, baking powder, and salt. In another bowl, whisk eggs, vanilla extract, almond milk, and melted coconut oil until well combined. Add the wet ingredients to the dry ingredients and mix until just combined. Gently fold in blueberries.

3. Baking: Divide the batter evenly among the muffin cups. Bake for 18-20 minutes until a toothpick inserted into the center comes out clean.

4. Serving: Let the muffins cool in the tin for 5 minutes, then transfer to a wire rack to cool completely.

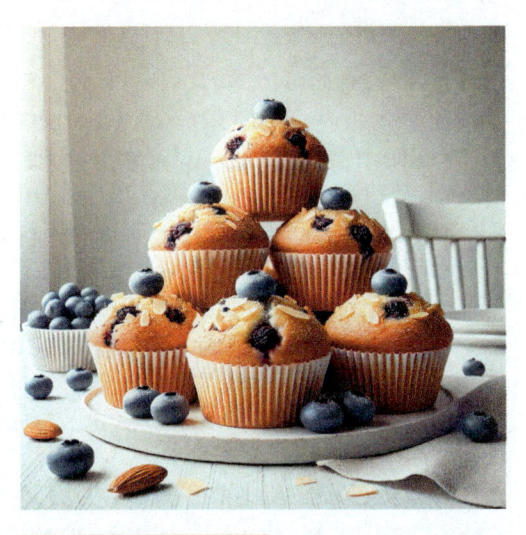

Nutritional Values: Calories: 150 kcal, Carbs: 8 g, Protein: 5 g, Fat: 12 g (Saturated Fat: 3 g, Monounsaturated Fat: 6 g, Polyunsaturated Fat: 2 g), Cholesterol: 55 mg, Sodium: 60 mg, Fiber: 3 g, Sugars: 7 g

Glycemic Index: Almond flour: Very Low (GI = 1), Blueberries: Low (GI = 53), Stevia: Very Low (GI = 0)

Chef's Tips: *"For added flavor, sprinkle the tops of the muffins with a few extra blueberries or a pinch of cinnamon before baking."*

89. Whole Wheat Banana Bread

Prep: 15 min | **Cook:** 50 min | **Total:** 1 hr 5 min | **Difficulty:** 2/5

Ingredients: Whole wheat flour: 1 1/2 cups (180g, 6.35 oz), Ripe bananas, mashed: 3 large (360g, 12.7 oz), Eggs: 2 large, Stevia: 1/4 cup (30g, 1.06 oz), Baking soda: 1 tsp (4g, 0.14 oz), Baking powder: 1/2 tsp (2g, 0.07 oz), Salt: 1/4 tsp (1g, 0.04 oz), Vanilla extract: 1 tsp (5 ml), Unsweetened almond milk: 1/4 cup (60 ml), Coconut oil: 1/4 cup (60 ml, 2.12 oz), Chopped walnuts (optional): 1/2 cup (50g, 1.76 oz)

1. Preparation: Preheat the oven to 350°F (175°C). Grease a loaf pan.
2. Mixing: Combine flour, baking soda, baking powder, and salt. Mix bananas, eggs, stevia, vanilla, almond milk, and coconut oil. Combine wet and dry ingredients. Fold in walnuts if using.
3. Baking: Pour batter into a loaf pan. Bake for 50-55 minutes until the toothpick comes out clean.
4. Serving: Cool in pan for 10 minutes, then transfer to a wire rack to cool completely before slicing.

Chef's Tips: *"For added flavor, sprinkle the top of the batter with a few extra chopped walnuts or a pinch of cinnamon before baking."*

Nutritional Values: Calories: 180 kcal, Carbs: 28 g, Protein: 4 g, Fat: 7 g (Saturated Fat: 2 g, Monounsaturated Fat: 3 g, Polyunsaturated Fat: 1 g), Cholesterol: 35 mg, Sodium: 150 mg, Fiber: 4 g, Sugars: 15 g (from bananas)

Glycemic Index: Whole wheat flour: Medium (GI = 69), Bananas: Medium (GI = 51), Stevia: Very Low (GI = 0)

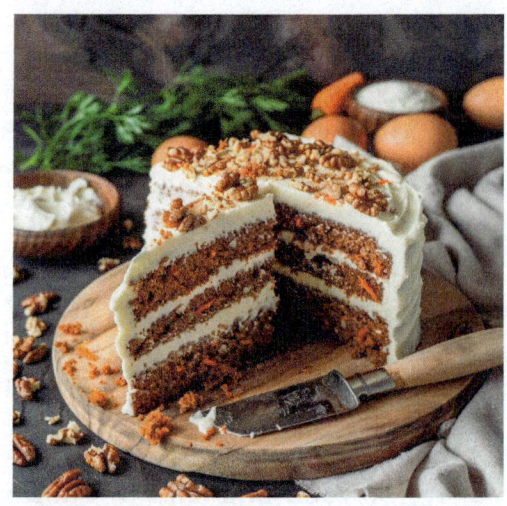

90. Carrot and Walnut Cake with Cream Cheese Frosting

Prep: 15 min | **Cook:** 30 min | **Total:** 45 min | **Difficulty:** 3/5

Ingredients: Whole wheat flour: 1 1/2 cups (180g), Baking powder: 1 tsp, Baking soda: 1 tsp, Ground cinnamon: 1 tsp, Ground nutmeg: 1/2 tsp, Salt: 1/4 tsp, Grated carrots: 1 1/2 cups (150g), Chopped walnuts: 1/2 cup (50g), Eggs: 2 large, Unsweetened applesauce: 1/2 cup (120ml), Plain Greek yogurt: 1/2 cup (120ml), Stevia: 1/4 cup (60ml), Vanilla extract: 1 tsp

Frosting: Light cream cheese: 1/2cup (120g), Plain Greek yogurt: 1/4cup (60ml), Stevia: 2 tbsp (30ml), Vanilla extract: 1/2tsp

1. Preparation: Preheat oven to 350°F (175°C), grease an 8-inch cake pan. Mix flour, baking powder, baking soda, cinnamon, nutmeg, and salt. Combine carrots and walnuts.
2. Mixing: Beat eggs, applesauce, yogurt, stevia, and vanilla. Add dry ingredients, fold in carrots and walnuts.
3. Baking: Pour batter into a cake pan. Bake for 25-30 minutes until the toothpick comes out clean.
4. Frosting: Beat cream cheese, yogurt, stevia, and vanilla. Spread over cooled cake.
5. Serving: Slice and serve, garnish with walnuts.

Nutritional Values: Calories: 200 kcal, Carbohydrates: 15g, Protein: 7g, Fat: 15g (Saturated Fat: 3g, Monounsaturated Fat: 4g, Polyunsaturated Fat: 6g), Cholesterol: 55mg, Sodium: 210mg, Fiber: 5g, Sugars: 15g

Glycemic Index: Whole wheat flour: Medium (GI = 69), Carrots: Medium (GI = 35-55), Walnuts: Low (GI = 15), Stevia: Very Low (GI = 0)

Chef's Tips: *"Add raisins or shredded coconut for extra flavor."*

91. Pumpkin Spice Bread

Prep: 15 min | **Cook:** 50 min | **Total:** 1 hr 5 min | **Difficulty:** 2/5
Ingredients: Whole wheat flour: 1 1/2 cups (180g, 6.35 oz), Pumpkin puree: 1 cup (240g, 8.47 oz), Eggs: 2 large, Stevia: 1/2 cup (60g, 2.12 oz), Baking soda: 1 tsp (4g, 0.14 oz), Baking powder: 1/2 tsp (2g, 0.07 oz), Salt: 1/4 tsp (1g, 0.04 oz), Pumpkin pie spice: 1 tsp (2g, 0.07 oz), Cinnamon: 1 tsp (2g, 0.07 oz), Vanilla extract: 1 tsp (5 ml), Unsweetened almond milk: 1/4 cup (60 ml), Coconut oil, melted: 1/4 cup (60 ml, 2.12 oz)
1. Preparation: Preheat the oven to 350°F (175°C). Grease a loaf pan.
2. Mixing: In a large bowl, whisk together whole wheat flour, baking soda, baking powder, salt, pumpkin pie spice, and cinnamon. In another bowl, mix pumpkin puree, eggs, stevia, vanilla extract, almond milk, and melted coconut oil until well combined. Add the wet ingredients to the dry ingredients and mix until just combined.
3. Baking: Pour batter into a loaf pan. Bake for 50-55 minutes until the toothpick comes out clean.
4. Serving: Let the pumpkin spice bread cool in the pan for 10 minutes, then transfer to a wire rack to cool completely before slicing.

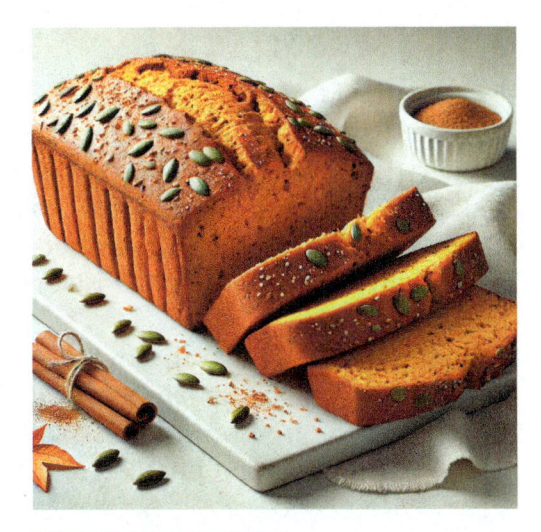

Nutritional Values: Calories: 160 kcal, Carbs: 28 g, Protein: 4 g, Fat: 6 g (Saturated Fat: 2 g, Monounsaturated Fat: 2 g, Polyunsaturated Fat: 1 g), Cholesterol: 35 mg, Sodium: 150 mg, Fiber: 4 g, Sugars: 9 g
Glycemic Index: Whole wheat flour: Medium (GI = 69), Pumpkin puree: Low (GI = 20), Stevia: Very Low (GI = 0)

Chef's Tips: *"For added flavor, sprinkle the top of the batter with a few extra pumpkin seeds or a pinch of cinnamon before baking."*

92. Oatmeal Raisin Cookies

Prep: 10 min | **Cook:** 15 min | **Total:** 25 min | **Difficulty:** 2/5
Ingredients: Rolled oats: 1 1/2 cups (150g, 5.29 oz), Whole wheat flour: 1 cup (120g, 4.23 oz), Raisins: 1/2 cup (75g, 2.65 oz), Stevia: 1/2 cup (60g, 2.12 oz), Baking soda: 1/2 tsp (2g, 0.07 oz), Cinnamon: 1 tsp (2g, 0.07 oz), Salt: 1/4 tsp (1g, 0.04 oz), Eggs: 2 large, Unsweetened applesauce: 1/2 cup (120g, 4.23 oz), Vanilla extract: 1 tsp (5 ml), Coconut oil, melted: 1/4 cup (60 ml, 2.12 oz)
1. Preparation: Preheat the oven to 350°F (175°C). Line a baking sheet with parchment paper.
2. Mixing: Mix oats, flour, baking soda, cinnamon, and salt. In another bowl, mix eggs, stevia, applesauce, vanilla, and coconut oil. Combine wet and dry ingredients. Fold in raisins.
3. Baking: Drop spoonfuls of dough onto a baking sheet, flatten slightly. Bake for 12-15 minutes until the edges are golden.
4. Serving: Cool on a baking sheet for 5 minutes, then transfer to a wire rack.

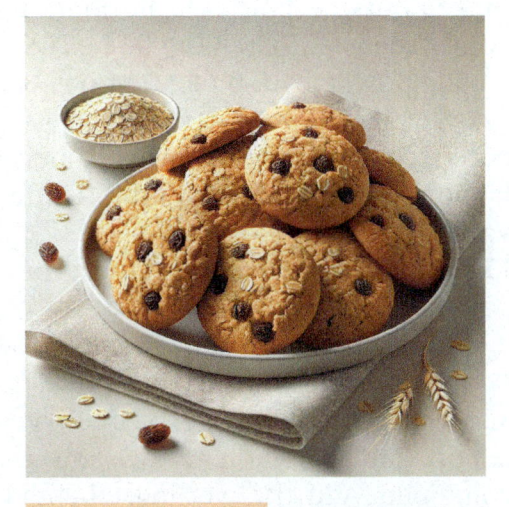

Nutritional Values: Calories: 120 kcal, Carbs: 22 g, Protein: 3 g, Fat: 4 g (Saturated Fat: 2 g, Monounsaturated Fat: 1 g, Polyunsaturated Fat: 1 g), Cholesterol: 15 mg, Sodium: 90 mg, Fiber: 3 g, Sugars: 19 g (from raisins)
Glycemic Index: Rolled oats: Medium (GI = 55), Whole wheat flour: Medium (GI = 69), Raisins: Medium (GI = 64), Stevia: Very Low (GI = 0)

Chef's Tips: *"For added flavor, add a handful of chopped nuts or a pinch of nutmeg to the dough before baking."*

93. Coconut Flour Brownies

Prep: 10 min | **Cook:** 25 min | **Total:** 35 min | **Difficulty:** 2/5
Ingredients: Coconut flour: 1/2 cup (60g, 2.12 oz), Cocoa powder: 1/2 cup (50g, 1.76 oz), Stevia: 1/2 cup (60g, 2.12 oz), Baking powder: 1/2 tsp (2g, 0.07 oz), Salt: 1/4 tsp (1g, 0.04 oz), Eggs: 4 large, Coconut oil, melted: 1/2 cup (120 ml, 4.23 oz), Vanilla extract: 1 tsp (5 ml), Unsweetened almond milk: 1/2 cup (120 ml)

1. **Preparation:** Preheat the oven to 350°F (175°C). Line an 8x8 inch (20x20 cm) baking pan with parchment paper.
2. **Mixing:** In a large bowl, whisk together coconut flour, cocoa powder, stevia, baking powder, and salt. In another bowl, whisk eggs, melted coconut oil, vanilla extract, and almond milk until well combined. Add the wet ingredients to the dry ingredients and mix until just combined.
3. **Baking:** Pour the batter into the prepared baking pan. Bake for 20-25 minutes until a toothpick inserted into the center comes out clean.
4. **Serving:** Let the brownies cool in the pan for 10 minutes, then transfer to a wire rack to cool completely before slicing.

Chef's Tips: *"For added flavor, fold in a handful of sugar-free chocolate chips or chopped nuts into the batter before baking."*

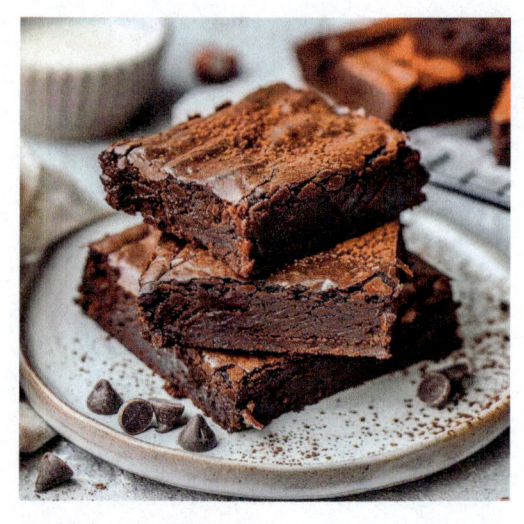

Nutritional Values: Calories: 180 kcal, Carbs: 10 g, Protein: 4 g, Fat: 14 g (Saturated Fat: 10 g, Monounsaturated Fat: 2 g, Polyunsaturated Fat: 1 g), Cholesterol: 80 mg, Sodium: 90 mg, Fiber: 4 g, Sugars: 4 g

Glycemic Index: Coconut flour: Very Low (GI = 45), Cocoa powder: Very Low (GI = 20), Stevia: Very Low (GI = 0)

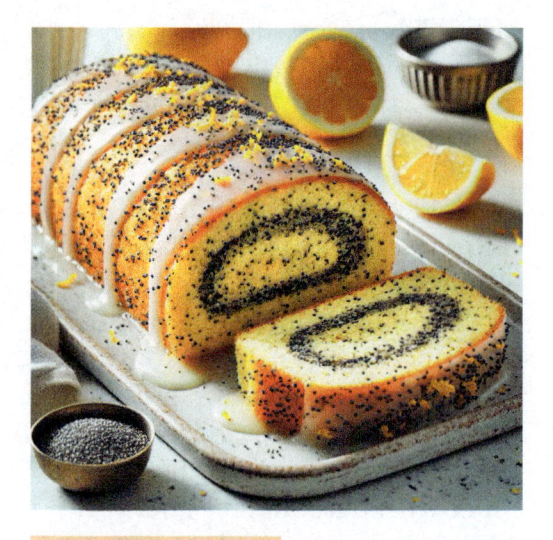

94. Lemon Poppy Seed Loaf

Prep: 15 min | **Cook:** 45 min | **Total:** 1 hr | **Difficulty:** 2/5
Ingredients: Whole wheat flour: 1 1/2 cups (180g, 6.35 oz), Poppy seeds: 2 tbsp (20g, 0.71 oz), Stevia: 1/2 cup (60g, 2.12 oz), Baking powder: 1 tsp (4g, 0.14 oz), Baking soda: 1/2 tsp (2g, 0.07 oz), Salt: 1/4 tsp (1g, 0.04 oz), Eggs: 2 large, Greek yogurt: 1/2 cup (120g, 4.23 oz), Coconut oil, melted: 1/4 cup (60 ml, 2.12 oz), Lemon juice: 1/4 cup (60 ml), Lemon zest: 1 tbsp (6g, 0.21 oz), Vanilla extract: 1 tsp (5 ml)

1. **Preparation:** Preheat the oven to 350°F (175°C). Grease a loaf pan.
2. **Mixing:** In a large bowl, whisk together whole wheat flour, poppy seeds, stevia, baking powder, baking soda, and salt. In another bowl, mix eggs, Greek yogurt, melted coconut oil, lemon juice, lemon zest, and vanilla extract until well combined. Add the wet ingredients to the dry ingredients and mix until just combined.
3. **Baking:** Pour the batter into the prepared pan. Bake for 40-45 minutes until a toothpick inserted into the center comes out clean.
4. **Serving:** Let the lemon poppy seed loaf cool in the pan for 10 minutes, then transfer to a wire rack to cool completely before slicing.

Chef's Tips: *"For added flavor, drizzle the loaf with a simple glaze made from lemon juice and stevia before serving."*

Nutritional Values: Calories: 180 kcal, Carbs: 25 g, Protein: 5 g, Fat: 7 g (Saturated Fat: 2 g, Monounsaturated Fat: 3 g, Polyunsaturated Fat: 1 g), Cholesterol: 35 mg, Sodium: 150 mg, Fiber: 4 g, Sugars: 5 g

Glycemic Index: Whole wheat flour: Medium (GI = 69), Greek yogurt: Low (GI = 30), Stevia: Very Low (GI = 0)

DESSERTS & SWEET TREATS

Special Treats

Note: These recipes are designed for one serving. To accommodate more people, simply multiply the ingredients by the desired number of servings.

The words "tablespoon" and "teaspoon" have been shortened to "tbsp" and "tsp".

95. Dark Chocolate Avocado Mousse

Prep: 10 min | **Cook:** 0 min | **Total:** 10 min | **Difficulty:** 1/5

Ingredients: Ripe avocados: 2 (300g, 10.58 oz), Unsweetened cocoa powder: 1/4 cup (30g, 1.06 oz), Dark chocolate (70% or higher), melted: 1/2 cup (100g, 3.53 oz), Stevia: 2 tbsp (8g, 0.28 oz), Vanilla extract: 1 tsp (5 ml), Almond milk: 1/4 cup (60 ml), Sea salt: a pinch

1. **Preparation:** Scoop the flesh from the avocados into a blender or food processor.
2. **Blending:** Add cocoa powder, melted dark chocolate, stevia, vanilla extract, almond milk, and sea salt. Blend until smooth and creamy.
3. **Chilling:** Transfer the mousse to serving bowls and refrigerate for at least 30 minutes before serving.
4. **Serving:** Garnish with fresh berries or a sprinkle of sea salt if desired.

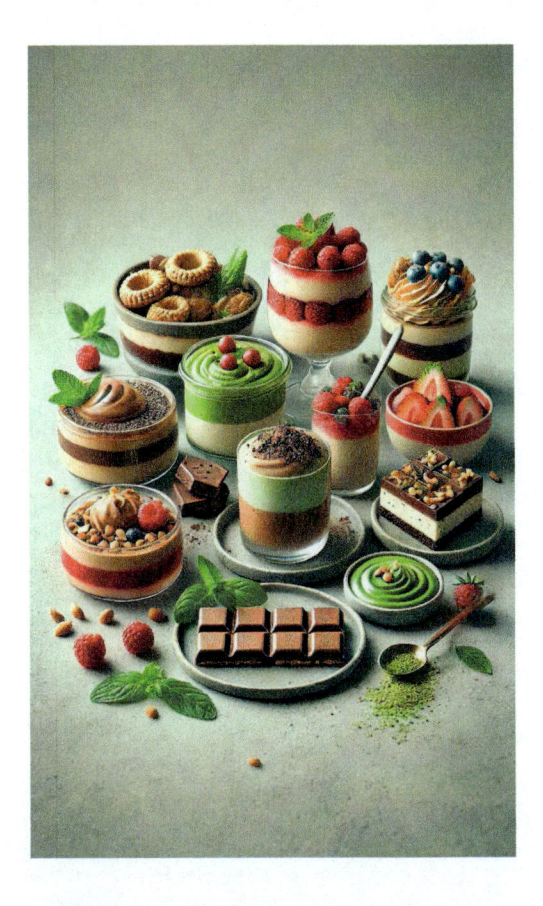

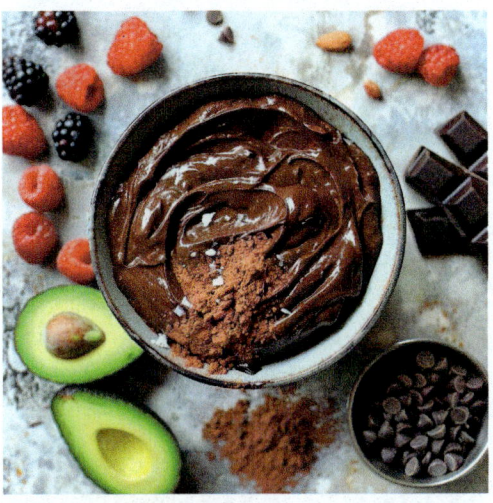

Nutritional Values: Calories: 200 kcal, Carbs: 18 g, Protein: 3 g, Fat: 15 g (Saturated Fat: 5 g, Monounsaturated Fat: 8 g, Polyunsaturated Fat: 2 g), Cholesterol: 0 mg, Sodium: 50 mg, Fiber: 8 g, Sugars: 3 g (from dark chocolate and almond milk)

Glycemic Index: Avocados: Very Low (GI = 15), Unsweetened cocoa powder: Very Low (GI = 20), Dark chocolate: Low (GI = 23), Stevia: Very Low (GI = 0)

Chef's Tips: *"For added texture, fold in some finely chopped nuts or a sprinkle of cacao nibs before chilling."*

96. Raspberry and Chia Seed Pudding

Prep: 5 min | **Cook:** 0 min | **Chill:** 4 hrs | **Total:** 4 hrs 5 min | **Difficulty:** 1/5

Ingredients: Chia seeds: 1/4 cup (50g, 1.76 oz), Unsweetened almond milk: 1 cup (240 ml), Stevia: 1 tsp (4g, 0.14 oz), Vanilla extract: 1 tsp (5 ml), Raspberries: 1 cup (150g, 5.29 oz), Fresh mint, chopped: 1 tbsp (4g, 0.14 oz)

1. **Preparation:** In a bowl, mix chia seeds, almond milk, stevia, and vanilla extract. Stir well to combine.
2. **Chilling:** Cover the bowl and refrigerate for at least 4 hours, or overnight, until the chia seeds have absorbed the liquid and the mixture has thickened.
3. **Serving:** Stir the chia pudding before serving. Top with raspberries and garnish with chopped fresh mint.

Chef's Tips: *"For added texture and flavor, sprinkle with a handful of granola or chopped nuts before serving."*

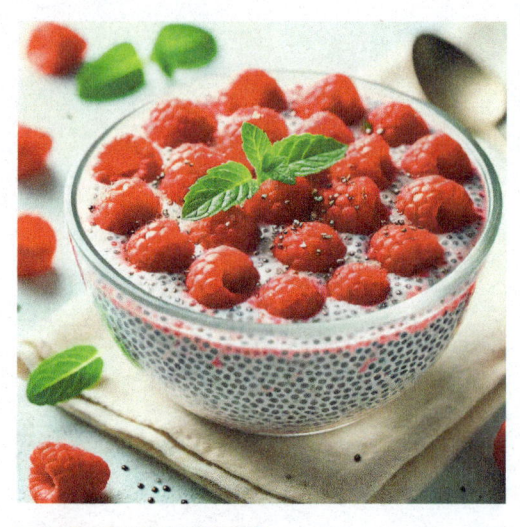

Nutritional Values: Calories: 150 kcal, Carbs: 18 g, Protein: 4 g, Fat: 7 g (Saturated Fat: 0.5 g, Monounsaturated Fat: 2 g, Polyunsaturated Fat: 4 g), Cholesterol: 0 mg, Sodium: 30 mg, Fiber: 8 g, Sugars: 5 g

Glycemic Index: Chia seeds: Very Low (GI = 1), Unsweetened almond milk: Very Low (GI = 30), Raspberries: Low (GI = 26)

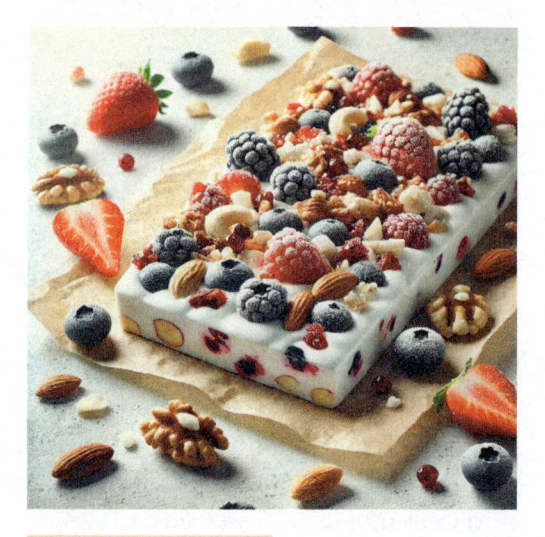

97. Frozen Yogurt Bark with Nuts and Berries

Prep: 10 min | **Cook:** 0 min | **Freeze:** 2 hrs | **Total:** 2 hrs 10 min | **Difficulty:** 1/5

Ingredients: Greek yogurt: 2 cups (480g, 16.93 oz), Stevia: 2 tbsp (8g, 0.28 oz), Mixed berries (strawberries, blueberries, raspberries): 1 cup (150g, 5.29 oz), Mixed nuts, chopped (almonds, walnuts, cashews): 1/2 cup (60g, 2.12 oz), Vanilla extract: 1 tsp (5 ml)

1. **Preparation:** Line a baking sheet with parchment paper.
2. **Mixing:** In a bowl, mix Greek yogurt, stevia, and vanilla extract until well combined.
3. **Assembly:** Spread the yogurt mixture evenly onto the prepared baking sheet. Sprinkle mixed berries and chopped nuts over the top.
4. **Freezing:** Place the baking sheet in the freezer and freeze for at least 2 hours, or until the yogurt is firm.
5. **Serving:** Break the frozen yogurt bark into pieces and serve immediately or store in the freezer until ready to eat.

Chef's Tips: *"For added flavor, sprinkle with shredded coconut before freezing."*

Nutritional Values: Calories: 180 kcal, Carbs: 15 g, Protein: 10 g, Fat: 8 g (Saturated Fat: 2 g, Monounsaturated Fat: 4 g, Polyunsaturated Fat: 2 g), Cholesterol: 5 mg, Sodium: 40 mg, Fiber: 3 g, Sugars: 8 g (from Greek yogurt and mixed berries)

Glycemic Index: Greek yogurt: Low (GI = 30), Mixed berries: Low (GI = 25), Mixed nuts: Very Low (GI = 15)

98. Coconut Macaroons

Prep: 10 min | **Cook:** 20 min | **Total:** 30 min | **Difficulty:** 2/5

Ingredients: Unsweetened shredded coconut: 2 cups (160g, 5.64 oz), Egg whites: 3 large, Stevia: 1/4 cup (30g, 1.06 oz), Vanilla extract: 1 tsp (5 ml), Salt: a pinch

1. **Preparation:** Preheat the oven to 325°F (160°C). Line a baking sheet with parchment paper.
2. **Mixing:** In a large bowl, combine shredded coconut, stevia, vanilla extract, and salt. In another bowl, beat egg whites until stiff peaks form. Gently fold the beaten egg whites into the coconut mixture until well combined.
3. **Baking:** Drop spoonfuls of the mixture onto the prepared baking sheet, spacing them about 2 inches apart. Bake for 18-20 minutes until the macaroons are golden brown on the edges.
4. **Serving:** Let the macaroons cool on the baking sheet for 5 minutes, then transfer to a wire rack to cool completely.

Chef's Tips: *"For added flavor, dip the bottoms of the cooled macaroons in melted dark chocolate and let them set on parchment paper."*

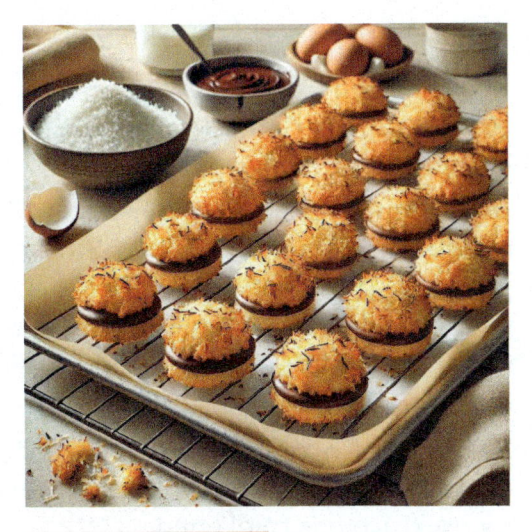

Nutritional Values: Calories: 120 kcal, Carbs: 6 g, Protein: 3 g, Fat: 10 g (Saturated Fat: 8 g, Monounsaturated Fat: 1 g, Polyunsaturated Fat: 0.5 g), Cholesterol: 0 mg, Sodium: 40 mg, Fiber: 4 g, Sugars: 0 g

Glycemic Index: Unsweetened shredded coconut: Very Low (GI = 10), Stevia: Very Low (GI = 0)

99. No-Bake Chocolate Peanut Butter Bars

Prep: 15 min | **Cook:** 0 min | **Chill:** 1 hr | **Total:** 1 hr 15 min | **Difficulty:** 2/5

Ingredients: Natural peanut butter: 1 cup (240g, 8.47 oz), Coconut flour: 1/2 cup (60g, 2.12 oz), Stevia: 1/4 cup (30g, 1.06 oz), Dark chocolate (70% or higher), melted: 1 cup (200g, 7.05 oz), Coconut oil: 1/4 cup (60 ml, 2.12 oz), Vanilla extract: 1 tsp (5 ml), Sea salt: a pinch

1. **Preparation:** Line an 8x8 inch (20x20 cm) baking dish with parchment paper.
2. **Mixing:** In a large bowl, mix peanut butter, coconut flour, stevia, vanilla extract, and a pinch of sea salt until well combined. Spread the mixture evenly into the prepared pan.
3. **Topping:** In a separate bowl, mix melted dark chocolate and coconut oil until smooth. Pour the chocolate mixture over the peanut butter layer, spreading it evenly.
4. **Chilling:** Refrigerate for at least 1 hour or until the bars are firm.
5. **Serving:** Cut into squares and serve. Store any leftovers in the refrigerator.

Chef's Tips: *"For added texture, sprinkle chopped nuts or a pinch of sea salt on top of the chocolate layer before chilling."*

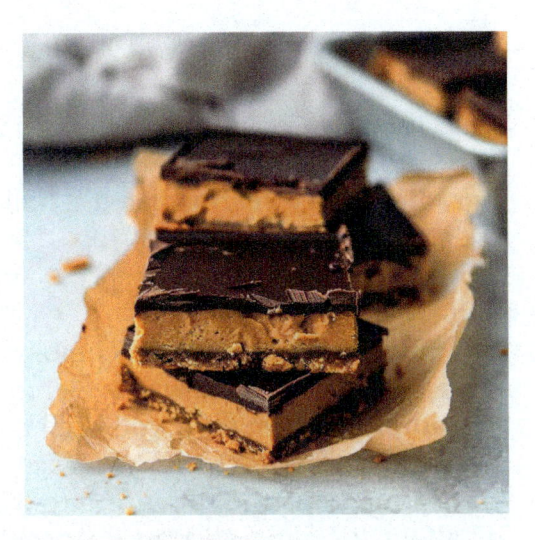

Nutritional Values: Calories: 250 kcal, Carbs: 12 g, Protein: 6 g, Fat: 20 g (Saturated Fat: 10 g, Monounsaturated Fat: 6 g, Polyunsaturated Fat: 2 g), Cholesterol: 0 mg, Sodium: 50 mg, Fiber: 5 g, Sugars: 3 g (from dark chocolate and almond milk)

Glycemic Index: Peanut butter: Low (GI = 14), Coconut flour: Very Low (GI = 45), Dark chocolate: Low (GI = 23), Stevia: Very Low (GI = 0)

100. Matcha Green Tea Pudding

Prep: 10 min | **Cook:** 0 min | **Chill:** 2 hrs | **Total:** 2 hrs 10 min | **Difficulty:** 1/5

Ingredients: Chia seeds: 1/4 cup (50g, 1.76 oz), Unsweetened almond milk: 1 cup (240 ml), Stevia: 1 tsp (4g, 0.14 oz), Matcha green tea powder: 1 tsp (2g, 0.07 oz), Vanilla extract: 1 tsp (5 ml)

1. Preparation: In a bowl, mix chia seeds, almond milk, stevia, matcha green tea powder, and vanilla extract. Stir well to combine.

2. Chilling: Cover the bowl and refrigerate for at least 2 hours, or overnight, until the chia seeds have absorbed the liquid and the mixture has thickened.

3. Serving: Stir the pudding before serving. Optionally, top with fresh berries or a sprinkle of coconut flakes.

Nutritional Values: Calories: 120 kcal, Carbs: 10 g, Protein: 4 g, Fat: 7 g (Saturated Fat: 0.5 g, Monounsaturated Fat: 2 g, Polyunsaturated Fat: 4 g), Cholesterol: 0 mg, Sodium: 30 mg, Fiber: 8 g, Sugars: 3 g

Glycemic Index: Chia seeds: Very Low (GI = 1), Unsweetened almond milk: Very Low (GI = 30), Matcha green tea powder: Very Low (GI = 0)

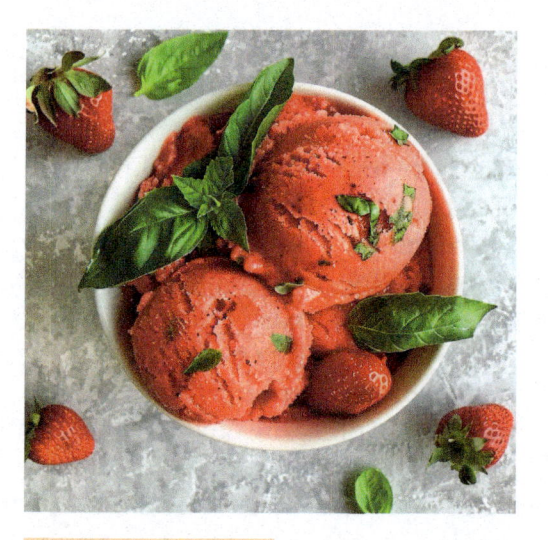

Chef's Tips: *"For added flavor, mix in a pinch of cinnamon or a few drops of almond extract."*

101. Strawberry Basil Sorbet

Prep: 10 min | **Cook:** 0 min | **Freeze:** 2 hrs | **Total:** 2 hrs 10 min | **Difficulty:** 2/5

Ingredients: Fresh strawberries, hulled: 4 cups (600g, 21.16 oz), Fresh basil leaves: 1/4 cup (10g, 0.35 oz), Stevia: 1/4 cup (30g, 1.06 oz), Lemon juice: 2 tbsp (30 ml, 1.01 oz), Water: 1/2 cup (120ml)

1. Preparation: In a blender, combine strawberries, basil leaves, stevia, lemon juice, and water. Blend until smooth.

2. Straining (optional): If you prefer a smoother texture, strain the mixture through a fine mesh sieve to remove seeds.

3. Freezing: Pour the mixture into a shallow container. Freeze for about 2 hours, stirring every 30 minutes to break up ice crystals.

4. Serving: Once fully frozen, scoop the sorbet into bowls and serve immediately.

Nutritional Values: Calories: 50 kcal, Carbs: 12 g, Protein: 1 g, Fat: 0 g (Saturated Fat: 0 g, Monounsaturated Fat: 0 g, Polyunsaturated Fat: 0 g), Cholesterol: 0 mg, Sodium: 0 mg, Fiber: 3 g, Sugars: 8 g (from strawberries and lemon juice)

Glycemic Index: Strawberries: Low (GI = 41), Stevia: Very Low (GI = 0)

Chef's Tips: *"For added flavor, garnish with fresh basil leaves or a splash of balsamic vinegar."*

Chapter 6: Your 30-Day Meal Plan

A well-structured meal plan is a powerful tool for managing diabetes and ensuring balanced nutrition daily. This 30-day plan provides detailed guides for breakfast, lunch, dinner, and snacks for monitoring and adjusting your diet to keep your blood sugar levels stable.

DAY	BREAKFAST	SNACK 1	LUNCH	SNACK 2	DINNER
1	7. Tomato and Basil Omelet (p.16)	67. Cucumber Slices with Hummus (p.51)	22. Grilled Chicken and Avocado Salad (p.25)	87. Blueberry Chia Pudding (p.62)	47. Cauliflower Curry with Chickpeas and Spinach (p.39)
2	21. Warm Cinnamon Chia Pudding (p.24)	88. Almond Flour Blueberry Muffins (p.63)	29. Turkey and Avocado Wrap with Spinach (p.29)	73. Edamame with Sea Salt (p.54)	59. Honey Mustard Glazed Chicken Thighs (p.46)
3	10. Strawberry Banana Smoothie (p.18)	80. Garlic Parmesan Roasted Asparagus (p.58)	36. Creamy Cauliflower and Leek Soup (p.33)	99. No-Bake Chocolate Peanut Butter Bars (p.69)	66. Chicken Alfredo with Zucchini Noodles (p.50)
4	1. Avocado Toast with Poached Egg (p.13)	68. Almond and Coconut Energy Balls (p.52)	33. Falafel and Hummus Wrap with Cucumber (p.31)	91. Pumpkin Spice Bread (p.65)	52. Tuna Steaks with Mango-Avocado Salsa (p.42)
5	15. Veggie - Packed Breakfast Burrito (p.21)	69. Apple Slices with Almond Butter (p.52)	27. Lentil and Feta Salad (p.28)	101. Strawberry Basil Sorbet (p.70)	61. Cauliflower Fried Rice with Chicken and Vegetables (p.48)
6	20. Mushroom and Spinach Frittata (p.24)	79. Roasted Sweet Potato Wedges (p.58)	25. Beet and Goat Cheese Salad (p.27)	85. Cinnamon Poached Pears (p.61)	55. Grilled Lemon Chicken with Quinoa and Kale Salad (p.44)
7	2. Greek Yogurt with Berries (p.14)	81. Baked Apples with Cinnamon and Walnuts (p.59)	40. Mushroom and Barley Soup (p.35)	74. Garlic and Herb Roasted Brussels Sprouts (p.55)	43. Stuffed Bell Peppers with Quinoa and Black Beans (p.37)
8	3. Oatmeal with Sliced Banana and Cinnamon (p.14)	89. Whole Wheat Banana Bread (p.64)	42. Zucchini and Fresh Herb Soup (p.36)	75. Quinoa Pilaf with Fresh Herbs (p.56)	53. Herb-Roasted Chicken with Root Vegetables (p.43)
9	12. Avocado and Berry Smoothie (p.19)	77. Balsamic Glazed Carrots (p.57)	26. Asian Chicken Salad with Sesame Dressing (p.27)	94. Lemon Poppy Seed Loaf (p.66)	49. Shrimp and Quinoa Paella (p.41)
10	18. Savory Oatmeal with Egg and Avocado (p.23)	70. Veggie Sticks with Guacamole (p.53)	23. Apple and Walnut Spinach Salad (p.26)	98. Coconut Macaroons (p.69)	50. Baked Cod with Herbed Tomatoes and Zucchini (p.41)

DAY	BREAKFAST	SNACK 1	LUNCH	SNACK 2	DINNER
11	4. Scrambled Eggs with Spinach and Mushrooms (p.15)	71. Whole Grain Crackers with Cream Cheese (p.53)	24. Taco Salad with Ground Turkey (p.26)	97. Frozen Yogurt Bark with Nuts and Berries (p.68)	60. Zucchini Noodles with Pesto and Cherry Tomatoes (p.47)
12	19. Warm Spiced Apples and Cottage Cheese (p.23)	76. Cauliflower Rice with Lemon and Parsley (p.56)	41. Butternut Squash and Apple Soup (p.36)	82. Mixed Berry Compote with Greek Yogurt (p.60)	44. Eggplant Parmesan with Spinach and Ricotta (p.38)
13	17. Zucchini Pancakes (p.22)	78. Green Bean Almondine (p.57)	37. Chicken and Quinoa Vegetable Soup (p.34)	92. Oatmeal Raisin Cookies (p.65)	48. Grilled Salmon with Asparagus and Lemon-Dill Sauce (p.40)
14	8. Berry Spinach Smoothie (p.17)	72. Berry and Nut Mix (p.54)	22. Grilled Chicken and Avocado Salad (p.25)	90. Carrot and Walnut Cake with Cream Cheese Frosting (p.64)	54. Turkey Meatballs in Tomato Basil Sauce (p.44)
15	5. Rye Bread with Smoked Salmon and Cream Cheese (p.15)	95. Dark Chocolate Avocado Mousse (p.67)	35. Mediterranean Veggie Wrap with Feta (p.32)	80. Garlic Parmesan Roasted Asparagus (p.58)	57. Pork Tenderloin with Apple and Sage (p.45)
16	14. Green Apple and Kale Smoothie (p.20)	68. Almond and Coconut Energy Balls (p.52)	30. Grilled Chicken Caesar Wrap (p.30)	83. Grilled Peaches with Honey and Mint (p.60)	46. Butternut Squash and Lentil Stew (p.39)
17	1. Avocado Toast with Poached Egg (p.13)	73. Edamame with Sea Salt (p.54)	32. Smoked Salmon and Cream Cheese Wrap (p.31)	86. Tropical Fruit Salad with Lime and Coconut (p.62)	58. Lamb Chops with Rosemary and Garlic (p.46)
18	9. Tropical Green Smoothie (p.18)	69. Apple Slices with Almond Butter (p.52)	40. Mushroom and Barley Soup (p.35)	84. Mango and Berry Parfait (p.61)	51. Scallops with Cauliflower Mash and Garlic Spinach (p.42)
19	15. Veggie-Packed Breakfast Burrito (p.21)	76. Cauliflower Rice with Lemon and Parsley (p.56)	25. Beet and Goat Cheese Salad (p.27)	96. Raspberry and Chia Seed Pudding (p.68)	56. Beef Stir-Fry with Bell Peppers and Snow Peas (p.45)
20	11. Peach and Kale Smoothie (p.19)	72. Berry and Nut Mix (p.54)	31. Black Bean and Corn Salsa Wrap (p.30)	100. Matcha Green Tea Pudding (p.70)	49. Shrimp and Quinoa Paella (p.41)
21	17. Zucchini Pancakes (p.22)	101. Strawberry Basil Sorbet (p.70)	24. Taco Salad with Ground Turkey (p.26)	80. Garlic Parmesan Roasted Asparagus (p.58)	63. Eggplant Lasagna with Ricotta and Mozzarella (p.49)

DAY	BREAKFAST	SNACK 1	LUNCH	SNACK 2	DINNER
22	2. Greek Yogurt with Berries (p.14)	75. Quinoa Pilaf with Fresh Herbs (p.56)	36. Creamy Cauliflower and Leek Soup (p.33)	94. Lemon Poppy Seed Loaf (p.66)	52. Tuna Steaks with Mango-Avocado Salsa (p.42)
23	10. Strawberry Banana Smoothie (p.18)	71. Whole Grain Crackers with Light Cream Cheese (p.53)	33. Falafel and Hummus Wrap with Cucumber (p.31)	81. Baked Apples with Cinnamon and Walnuts (p.59)	59. Honey Mustard Glazed Chicken Thighs (p.46)
24	15. Veggie-Packed Breakfast Burrito (p.21)	68. Almond and Coconut Energy Balls (p.52)	22. Grilled Chicken and Avocado Salad (p.25)	99. No-Bake Chocolate Peanut Butter Bars (p.69)	64. Stuffed Portobello Mushrooms with Spinach and Feta (p.49)
25	64. Stuffed Portobello Mushrooms with Spinach and Feta (p.49)	77. Balsamic Glazed Carrots (p.57)	41. Butternut Squash and Apple Soup (p.36)	85. Cinnamon Poached Pears (p.61)	43. Stuffed Bell Peppers with Quinoa and Black Beans (p.37)
26	21. Warm Cinnamon Chia Pudding (p.24)	67. Cucumber Slices with Hummus (p.51)	29. Turkey and Avocado Wrap with Spinach (p.29)	89. Whole Wheat Banana Bread (p.64)	65. Cauliflower Crust Pizza with Veggie Toppings (p.50)
27	14. Green Apple and Kale Smoothie (p.20)	95. Dark Chocolate Avocado Mousse (p.67)	26. Asian Chicken Salad with Sesame Dressing (p.27)	79. Roasted Sweet Potato Wedges (p.58)	50. Baked Cod with Herbed Tomatoes and Zucchini (p.41)
28	5. Rye Bread with Smoked Salmon and Cream Cheese (p.15)	82. Mixed Berry Compote with Greek Yogurt (p.60)	25. Beet and Goat Cheese Salad (p.27)	70. Veggie Sticks with Guacamole (p.53)	61. Cauliflower Fried Rice with Chicken and Vegetables (p.48)
29	7. Tomato and Basil Omelet (p.16)	76. Cauliflower Rice with Lemon and Parsley (p.56)	30. Grilled Chicken Caesar Wrap (p.30)	86. Tropical Fruit Salad with Lime and Coconut (p.62)	62. Spaghetti Squash Bolognese (p.48)
30	20. Mushroom and Spinach Frittata (p.24)	78. Green Bean Almondine (p.57)	32. Smoked Salmon and Cream Cheese Wrap (p.31)	88. Almond Flour Blueberry Muffins (p.63)	53. Herb-Roasted Chicken with Root Vegetables (p.43)

These adaptations ensure that everyone can enjoy delicious, diabetes-friendly meals, regardless of dietary restrictions.

Appendix A: Glycemic Index Chart

The Glycemic Index (GI) is a useful tool for managing diabetes. This chart lists common foods and their GI values to help you make informed dietary choices.

GI CATEGORY	GI RANGE	EXAMPLE FOODS
Low GI	55 or less	Apples, barley, lentils, milk, peanuts, chickpeas, strawberries, carrots, sweet corn, quinoa
Medium GI	56-69	Brown rice, whole wheat bread, sweet potatoes, pineapple, oatmeal, couscous, bananas, beets, bulgur, grapes
High GI	70 or more	White bread, rice cakes, watermelon, cornflakes, instant mashed potatoes, pretzels, jasmine rice, doughnuts, parsnips, glucose

Appendix B: Micronutrient Table

MICRONUTRIENT	FUNCTION	FOOD SOURCES
Vitamin A	Supports vision, immune system, and reproductive health.	Carrots, spinach, sweet potatoes, liver, eggs.
Vitamin B1 (Thiamin)	Helps convert nutrients into energy.	Whole grains, pork, seeds, nuts, legumes.
Vitamin B2 (Riboflavin)	Important for growth, energy production, and the breakdown of fats.	Milk, eggs, almonds, spinach, chicken.
Vitamin B3 (Niacin)	Helps convert food into energy and maintains healthy skin and nerves.	Chicken, turkey, salmon, whole wheat, avocados.
Vitamin B5 (Pantothenic Acid)	Aids in the synthesis of fatty acids and the metabolism of proteins and carbohydrates.	Chicken, beef, potatoes, oats, tomatoes.
Vitamin B6 (Pyridoxine)	Important for protein metabolism, cognitive development, and immune function.	Chickpeas, bananas, salmon, chicken, potatoes.
Vitamin B7 (Biotin)	Helps with energy metabolism and supports healthy hair, skin, and nails.	Eggs, almonds, spinach, sweet potatoes, cheese.
Vitamin B9 (Folate)	Essential for cell division and the formation of DNA and RNA.	Leafy greens, legumes, avocados, oranges, seeds.
Vitamin B12 (Cobalamin)	Necessary for red blood cell formation, neurological function, and DNA synthesis.	Fish, meat, poultry, eggs, dairy products.
Vitamin C	Antioxidant that supports immune function and collagen synthesis.	Oranges, strawberries, bell peppers, kiwi, broccoli.
Vitamin D	Important for calcium absorption and bone health.	Fatty fish, egg yolks, fortified foods, sun exposure.

Vitamin E	Antioxidant that helps protect cells from damage.	Almonds, sunflower seeds, spinach, avocados, sweet potatoes.
Vitamin K	Essential for blood clotting and bone health.	Leafy greens, broccoli, Brussels sprouts, cabbage, fish.
Calcium	Important for bone health and muscle function.	Dairy products, fortified plant-based milks, leafy greens, tofu.
Iron	Essential for oxygen transport in the blood and muscle function.	Red meat, poultry, legumes, spinach, quinoa.
Magnesium	Important for muscle and nerve function, blood sugar control, and energy production.	Almonds, spinach, black beans, avocado, whole grains.
Phosphorus	Supports the formation of bones and teeth and is involved in energy metabolism.	Dairy products, salmon, chicken, nuts, whole grains.
Potassium	Helps maintain normal blood pressure, supports nerve and muscle function.	Bananas, oranges, potatoes, spinach, avocados.
Zinc	Supports immune function, wound healing, and DNA synthesis.	Meat, shellfish, legumes, seeds, nuts.
Selenium	Antioxidant that plays a role in DNA synthesis and protects against infection.	Brazil nuts, seafood, meat, eggs, brown rice.
Copper	Important for iron metabolism, energy production, and brain function.	Shellfish, nuts, seeds, whole grains, dark chocolate.
Manganese	Involved in the metabolism of amino acids, cholesterol, and carbohydrates.	Whole grains, nuts, legumes, leafy greens, tea.
Fluoride	Helps prevent dental cavities.	Fluoridated water, tea, seafood.
Iodine	Essential for the production of thyroid hormones.	Iodized salt, seafood, dairy products, seaweed.

Appendix C: Resources for Further Reading

Expand your knowledge and stay informed with these recommended resources:
- **Books:**
    - "The Diabetes Code" by Dr. Jason Fung
    - "The Diabetes Solution" by Dr. Richard Bernstein
- **Websites:**
    - American Diabetes Association (www.diabetes.org)
    - Mayo Clinic (www.mayoclinic.org)
- **Support Groups:**
    - DiabetesSisters (www.diabetessisters.org)
    - JDRF (www.jdrf.org)

Thanks for reading my book! I hope you found it helpful. If you have a moment, I'd love to hear your thoughts. Your review can help other readers discover my work. Thanks a lot for your support!

MOIRA BOYD

Printed in Great Britain
by Amazon